Infection Control

Infection Control

HOSPITAL AND COMMUNITY

Claire Mercier

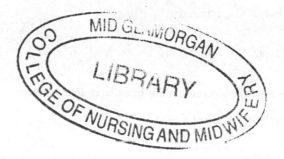

Stanley Thornes (Publishers) Ltd

© 1997 Claire Mercier

The right of Claire Mercier to be identified as author of this work has been asserted by her in accordance with the Copyright, Designs and Patents Act 1988.

All rights reserved. No part of this publication may be reproduced or transmitted in any form or by any means, electronic or mechanical, including photocopying, recording or any information storage and retrieval system, without permission in writing from the publisher or under licence from the Copyright Licensing Agency Limited. Further details of such licences (for reprographic reproduction) may be obtained from the Copyright Licensing Agency Limited, of 90 Tottenham Court Road, London W1P 9HE.

First published in 1997 by:
Stanley Thornes (Publishers) Ltd
Ellenborough House
Wellington Street
CHELTENHAM
GL50 1YW
United Kingdom

97 98 99 00 01 / 10 9 8 7 6 5 4 3 2 1

A catalogue record for this book is available from the British Library

ISBN 0-7487-3319-1

Typeset by Acorn Bookwork, Salisbury, Wilts.
Printed and bound in Great Britain by TJ International, Padstow, Cornwall

Contents

Preface

This book has been written as an infection control guide for all health care professionals working in hospitals and in the community. In hospitals, it is addressed to medical, nursing, physiotherapy and occupational therapy staff. In the community, it is for general practitioners, dentists, practice nurses and nursing and residential home staff.

Staff can only follow good infection control practice if they understand what they are doing. Many current infection control practices are still based on ritual and tradition rather than research. The reason I wrote this book is that, while giving infection control advice in both hospital and the community, I felt that there was a need for a book which explained infection control practice simply but fully. I hope that I have achieved this.

Acknowledgements

I would like to thank everyone who helped me to write this book. In particular Janet Howard who has been nothing short of brilliant with her ideas, timing and the amount of hard work she put in. Chris Evennett who, among other things, has helped enormously with keeping me up to date with the NHS reforms, David Wright who pointed me in the right direction, Iain Templeton who offered some very constructive criticism and Tony Ellam for his contribution. I would also like to thank all my colleagues over the past three years who have answered my many questions as I've gone along.

Finally I would like to dedicate this book to my parents, thank you both so much for all your love and support.

Historical background to infection control

Infection and its prevention have been a prime concern of mankind for a long time. Hospitals have been in existence to care for the sick and dying since 500 BC. At this time those provided by the Ancient Jews depended on the literal application of the Old Testament laws found in Leviticus. The cleanliness associated with these early hospitals was based on religious beliefs of purity, rather than any understanding of cross-infection. After the decline of the Roman Empire, hygiene standards, including hospital hygiene, fell throughout Europe. Christianity undertook to heal the sick, and the church monopolised early medical practice with priests having the privilege of the cure of bodies as well as that of souls (Poynter, 1964). Unfortunately the early Christian Church was opposed to washing and conditions in medieval hospitals were very poor. Infection in hospital, particularly of wounds was extremely common in the middle ages. The majority of medical practitioners at this time believed that 'laudable pus' was a prerequisite for wound healing. Some doctors would even take pus from an infected wound of a patient and place it on the clean wound of another in the belief that this would help it heal. Early pioneers who disagreed were persecuted (Major, 1954). Most hospitals of the period were overcrowded, with two or more patients to every bed, and there was a prevailing foul odour. It was mainly the poor and homeless who used these institutions, and the majority died. Wealthier people were nursed in their own homes.

While it was becoming obvious that the majority of patients in hospitals died, the problem of infection spreading in the community was also causing concern. Major epidemics were common, for example plague, cholera and typhoid.

DEVELOPMENT OF HOSPITAL INFECTION CONTROL

During wars, from as far back as the eighteenth century, large numbers of soldiers, who survived death on the battle field, lost their lives to wound infections later and this had very serious military consequences. Due to the high mortality associated with military hospitals, a number of significant advances in hospital infection control were instigated. In 1740, a hundred years before Florence Nightingale made her observations in Scutari, a physician to the British army, Sir John Pringle, introduced sanitary reforms in an effort to improve the health of the forces. Pringle observed that military hospitals were among the chief causes of sickness and death in the army. He also observed that infection was 'the common and fatal consequence of a large and crowded hospital' (Pringle, 1752). Many of these military hospital inpatients did not die as a result of their wounds but from epidemics of louse-borne typhus and dysentery (Cantile, 1974).

Typhus, or jail fever, also had a high mortality rate among previously healthy individuals. In 1750, an outbreak occurred which was centred on the Old Bailey courts; the Lord Mayor, the judges, and many jury members and others in court all died from the disease.

As with so many infection control problems, puerperal fever, a disease associated with mortality after childbirth was a hospital problem, caused by cross-infection due to poor, if not non-existent, hand hygiene. In the Vienna General Hospital there were two obstetric clinics. Medical students were taught in one and midwives in the second. The death rate in the clinic training the medical students was far higher (10%) than the clinic training midwives (3%) (Semmelweis, 1861). Semmelweis set out to investigate this. Following the introduction in the late 1840s, of chlorinated lime to deodorise, but which also unintentionally disinfected hands, he observed a tenfold reduction in the incidence of puerperal fever.

In the nineteenth century the long-held concept of infection emanating from the environment began to gain scientific support. This knowledge of infection was incorporated into medical knowledge by doctors, such as Joseph Lister, who used carbolic spray on cotton wool applied to wounds to help prevent surgical wound infections. He was later to accept that his success was due more to the spray landing on and disinfecting hands, instruments and sutures, rather than the wound dressing itself.

However, despite the credence being given to the new scientific knowledge, it took some time for the information to filter through to the medical establishment. Florence Nightingale was a great believer in the importance of cleanliness, fresh air, space and light to banish disease. The design of many of the hospitals built in the latter half of the nineteenth century was as a direct consequence of her beliefs. She also introduced the concept of 'fever nursing'. By the end of the nineteenth century much work had been done on nosocomial infection, with the aim of minimising the risk of hospital acquired infection.

IMPROVEMENTS IN COMMUNITY INFECTION CONTROL

The dramatic changes in the incidence of many infectious diseases which have occurred in the last two centuries have been brought about by many factors; the provision of a clean water supply, effective sewage disposal and the reduction of overcrowding through better living conditions. These have always been essential prerequisites for effective control, and contributed to a reduction in incidence long before the introduction of modern medicine. An example of this is that the incidence of diseases such as tuberculosis began to decline, long before the introduction of effective antibiotics. Improvements in nutrition and effective health education have also played their role.

INFECTION CONTROL IN THE TWENTIETH CENTURY

During the twentieth century scientific knowledge has increased tremendously, with most school children having a greater understanding of infection than the great men of science 100 years ago. The means of treating infections in both the hospital and the community has increased dramatically worldwide. There have been two major advances in the prevention and treatment of infectious diseases. The most important has been the progressive development of vaccines against rubella, measles, diphtheria and whooping cough which has culminated in the global eradication of smallpox and is expected to eliminate poliomyelitis by the year 2005. The second advance has been the development of antibiotics since the 1940s; thus, dramatically reducing mortality rates previously associated with many common fatal diseases such as pneumonia, tuberculosis, and many of the common childhood diseases.

Regrettably this increased understanding of hospital acquired infection (HAI) has not always been matched with a wiser use of the resources at our disposal. The largely uncontrolled use of antibiotics in the hospital environment and poor prescribing in the community has led inexorably and inevitably to the development of multi-drug resistant organisms.

Present day problems

Diseases are continuing to flourish and cause infection both in the hospital and the community. We have created our own twentieth century infection problems with organisms that are resistant to many antibiotics, e.g. methicillin resistant *Staphylococcus aureus* (MRSA) (Marples and Reith, 1992), and vancomycin resistant enterococci (VRE). These are a problem for hospitals and require containment measures (*J. Hosp. Infect.*, 1990; HICPAC, 1995). In the community, infections may also be spread in nursing and residential homes, homes for people with learning disabilities, schools and nurseries, guidelines have been written for these areas (Chouillet, 1992; Ross, 1993). People who come into hospitals with infections, e.g. pneumococcal pneumonia and urinary tract infections (UTIs) can be the source of nosocomial infection outbreaks. The medical profession and general public can no longer rely solely on treating organisms with antibiotics; we need to concentrate again on the basics: proven infection control procedures. This concept has been reinforced by the appearance of new diseases for which no effective treatment or vaccines are available, e.g. human immunodeficiency virus (HIV) and hepatitis C virus (HCV). These diseases have forced us to refocus infection control practice on preventing the spread of infection by using control measures which include:

- surveillance of infections;
- prophylaxis/treatment;
- universal infection control precautions;
- immunisation.

Surveillance of infection

Surveillance is an essential component of the prevention and control of infection in the hospital and in the community. It involves the collection of data on infections among the population, analysis of the data and dissemination of the resulting information to the health care workers who can take appropriate action. Surveillance, in the very crudest terms, could be said to have begun in England in the fourteenth century, as Edward I kept a record of people with leprosy so that they could be expelled from the city of London. England can also claim to be one of the first countries in the world to keep a record of deaths; these were the Bills of Mortality, which began in the sixteenth century. One of the purposes they served was to enable the Court to leave the City of London for the then rural safety of Windsor when plague was rife.

Today the two main objectives of surveillance are:

- the prevention and early detection of outbreaks in the hospital and community;
- the assessment of infection levels over time in order to audit the effectiveness of infection control and prevention measures.

A wide variety of surveillance methods are used in the UK at present. The prevalence/incidence of hospital acquired infection is now often seen as a quality indicator, and more and more hospitals are beginning to look at their infection rates. Work is also being undertaken countrywide.

Prophylaxis and treatment

Current medical practice has adopted a strategy for minimising infection risks by the use of antibiotics given prophylactically prior to operative procedures. When first available, indiscriminate use of prophylactic antibiotics contributed to the emergence of multiple resistance in hospital bacteria and lead to an uncritical condemnation of the practice. Properly conducted trials have since conclusively demonstrated the value of prophylactic antibiotics in the following procedures: bowel surgery, hip or knee replacement operations, heart transplant operations, and dental procedures in patients with endocardial disease.

Treatment with antibiotics, antifungicidals and antiviral agents requires a co-ordinated approach to chemotherapy which can only be provided through a comprehensive written drugs policy involving all members of the multidisciplinary team, in both the hospital and the community. Antibiotics have been one of the most important medical advances of the twentieth century. Now that mechanisms of resistance are understood we need to use them wisely so that they can continue to be used effectively in the twenty-first century.

Universal infection control precautions

Blood and body fluids may contain blood borne viruses (e.g. hepatitis B, C and HIV) or other bacterial and viral pathogens and therefore present a risk to patients and staff. As it is not always possible to know who is infected with these pathogens, there are infection control precautions which must be taken with all blood and body fluids at all times. This practice which has been described as universal infection control precautions (UICP), but which is also known as body substance isolation (BSI) is based on the concept of risk assessment of the potential exposure to these fluids.

UICP contains the following components:

- handwashing;
- protective clothing;
- safe handling and disposal of sharps and spillages;
- isolation procedures;
- other infection control policies including the disposal of waste, laundry, disinfection and sterilisation should also be based on UICP.

Handwashing

Handwashing is the single most important measure in infection control, (Reybrouck, 1983; Larson, 1994; Jarvis, 1994). Health care workers

(HCWs) should understand when and how to wash their hands, as well as being provided with adequate facilities to carry out the procedure.

Cuts and abrasions on the hands and arms should be covered with waterproof plasters.

Protective clothing

The use of protective clothing (gloves, aprons and eye/face protection) must be based on a risk assessment. If the health care worker feels that when they perform a certain task or procedure they will or may come into contact with blood or body fluids, then the appropriate protective clothing must be worn.

Disposable gloves must be worn if the health care worker anticipates direct contact with blood or body fluids and also if they are going to have direct contact with non-intact skin or mucous membranes. Gloves must always be discarded and the hands washed after each procedure. While wearing protective clothing to protect themselves, HCWs must not forget that using the same gloves for each client contact can lead to cross-infection (Vickers et al., 1994).

Disposable aprons should be worn whenever contamination of clothing with blood or body fluid is anticipated.

Eye/face protection must be worn during any procedure when there is a risk of blood or body fluid splashing onto the face.

Safe handling and disposal of sharps

A sharp is any item which is capable of penetrating or cutting the skin (e.g. needles, scalpels, stitch cutters and glass slides). All used sharps must be placed into a rigid sharps container complying to UN3291 (formerly British Standards 7320; BSI, 1990) immediately after use. Needles should never be bent or broken and resheathing needles (MDD, 1993) should be avoided whenever possible but, if necessary, a single handed scoop method must be adopted. Discard the needle and syringe as one unit into a sharps container. Keep the sharps container in a safe place, out of the reach of children (BMA, 1990). Never fill the sharps container more than three quarters full, and ensure that it is securely closed (DoH, 1993) and labelled with the source of origin before disposal as clinical waste.

A sharps injury policy must be in place. All sharps injuries must be recorded (HSE, 1993). A Hepatitis B immunisation policy for staff who undertake exposure prone procedures must be in place and operational.

Spillages

Spillages of blood or body fluid which is visibly stained with blood must be dealt with immediately. They should be treated with chlorine granules (e.g. Presept) and disposable gloves and an apron should be worn. There is commercial equipment available on the market to minimise the hazard associated with clearing up blood spillages. Spillages of other body substances, such as urine, faeces and vomit should be absorbed onto disposable towels/wipes and then discarded into yellow waste bags.

Isolation procedures

Isolating patients in hospitals is still common practice. In an ideal world if UICPs were followed at all times (hands washed and protective clothing worn), and if all patients in hospitals were cared for in well designed single rooms there would rarely be a need to segregate people in hospitals by placing them in isolation. Unfortunately most hospitals in the UK do not have many single rooms, and therefore patient isolation is still practised as a form of infection control. However, the effectiveness of the current isolation precautions are coming under scrutiny as the number of people with multi-drug resistant organisms increases. Outbreaks of multi-drug resistant tuberculosis (MDRTB) have occurred in the UK as well as the USA, and the need for additional precautions such as negative pressure rooms is now recognised.

Immunisation

The practice of immunisation is known to be one of the most cost effective medical practices. Outstanding examples are the global elimination of smallpox and major reductions in the incidence of measles, diphtheria, poliomyelitis and whooping cough in the western world. Unfortunately in many parts of the world, such as Africa and India, many childhood illnesses for which there are effective immunisations still cause serious morbidity and mortality. The World Health Organisation (WHO) is committed to eradicating poliomyelitis, caused by wild strains of the virus, by the year 2005. It has also set itself objectives to reduce the incidence of other childhood illnesses, such as measles, worldwide. In many countries this is being achieved through national immunisation days, when all children within a certain age-group are immunised over a very short period of time. In 1995, in China 80 000 000 children were immunised in one day. This type of commitment, which is costly for the country undertaking the programme who are generally the poorer countries in the world, will hopefully reduce the number of children worldwide dying unnecessarily from infectious diseases.

In the hospital, hepatitis B immunisation of health care workers perceived to be at risk has reduced the incidence of occupationally acquired hepatitis B to that of the general population in the USA. Following a number of outbreaks of hepatitis B in the UK associated with cardiothoracic and obstetric surgery, the Department of Health issued guidelines requiring the immune status of relevant health care

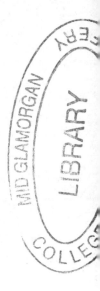

workers to be documented and those undertaking exposure-prone procedures to be immunised.

In the UK, HCWs providing maternity care should be known to be immune to rubella and if susceptible, immunised. Although a vaccine for chickenpox is not licensed in the UK, HCWs caring for HIV-positive and other immunocompromised patients should have their immune status documented so that prompt action to prevent unnecessary exposure of immunocompromised patients to chickenpox can be taken.

For many years the UK has depended on the use of BCG as a primary element in the control of tuberculosis. National recommendations promote the use of BCG in HCWs, particularly those working with susceptible groups, e.g. paediatrics, maternity and the immunocompromised.

THE FUTURE

Most work on cross infection in the eighteenth and nineteenth century concentrated on the hospital, whereas now that we are moving into the twenty-first century we are beginning to focus on the community. In the 1990s patients are transferred home from hospital much earlier than they were even in the mid-1980s, and many more operations are being carried out on a day care basis. Other minor invasive procedures are being performed regularly in the community. The widespread use of antibiotics has lead to multi-drug resistant organisms, and the resurgence of tuberculosis and multi-drug resistant tuberculosis has lead many health care workers to question the infection control precautions currently practised and to insist that infection control practice is based on evidence and research. A basic understanding of micro-organisms, the roles of the infection control practitioners and the concept of universal infection control precautions should enable the health care worker, whether based in the hospital or community, to be able to practise their chosen profession both safely and efficiently.

REFERENCES

British Medical Association (1990) *A Code of Practice for the Safe Use and Disposal of Sharps*, BMA. London.

British Standards Institute (1990) *Specification for sharps containers*, BS7320.

Cantile, N. (1974) *A History of the Army Medical Department,* volume 1, Churchill Livingstone, London.

Centres for Disease Control and Prevention (1994) *Preventing the Spread of Vancomycin Resistance – Report from the Hospital Infection Control Practices*

Advisory Committee; Comment Period and Public Meeting Notice. Federal Register, May 17, **59**: 25757–63. *CDCP Tech. Rep.*

Chouillet, A. (1992) Policies for control of communicable disease in day care centres. *Archives of Childhood Disease*, **67**, 1103–6.

Department of Health (1993) *Use and Management of Sharps Containers*, SAB(93)53, Department of Health, London.

Health and Safety Executive (1993) Needlestick Injuries. HSE information sheet. *HSE Tech. Rep. 1993.*

HICPAC (1995) Recommendations for preventing the spread of vancomycin resistance: recommendations of the Hospital Infection Control Practices Advisory Committeee (HICPAC). *American Journal of Infection Control*, **23**, 87–94.

Jarvis, W.R. (1994) Handwashing – the Semmelweis lesson forgotten? *Lancet*, **344** (8933) 1311–12.

Journal of Hospital Infection (1990) Report of the combined working party of the Hospital Infection Society and British Society for Antimicrobial Chemotherapy. Revised guidelines for the control of epidemic methicillin resistant *Staphylococcus aureus. Journal of Hospital Infection* **16**, 351–77.

Larson, E.L. (1994) Guidelines for handwashing and hand antiseptics in health care settings. *APIC*, **22** (5), 25A–47A.

Major, R.H. (1954) *A History of Medicine*, volume 1, Blackwell, Oxford pp. 294–321.

Marples, R.R. and Reith, S. (1992) Methicillin resistant *Staphylococcus aureus* in England and Wales. *CDR Review*, **2** (3), R25–29.

Medical Devices Directorate (1993) Resheathing needles after use and improper disposal. HAZ(93)11. *Medical Devices Directorate Tech. Rep. 8 April 1993.*

Poynter, F.N.L. (1964) *The Evolution of Hospitals in Britain*, Pitman Medical Publishing Company Ltd, London .

Pringle, J. (1752) *Observations on the Diseases of the Army, in Camp and Garrison*, Miller Wilson and Payne, London.

Reybrouck, G. (1983) Role of the hands in the spread of nosocomial infections. *Journal of Hospital Infection*, **4**, 103–10.

Ross, S. (1993) Creche Course. How to ensure hygiene in day nurseries. *Nursing Times Journal of Infection Control Nursing*, **89**, (29) 1–6.

Semmelweis, I.P. (1861) *Die Aetiologie, der Begriff, und die Prophylaxis des Kindbettfiebers*, Pest, Wein U., Leipzig.

Vickers, J., Painter, M.J., Heptonstall, J., Yusof, J.H.M. and Craske, J. (1994) Hepatitis B outbreak in a drug trials unit; investigation and recommendations. *CDR Review*, **4**(1), R1–R4.

2 | The microbiology laboratory and specimen collection

In the modern health care system, sending specimens off to the laboratory is seen as a normal and routine procedure. Indeed hospitals rely very heavily on the work of the laboratory. However many HCWs are unsure of what happens to specimens once they have been taken and sent to the laboratory. The following is a brief overview of the laboratory and the roles of the personnel who work there. In the laboratory, there are the clerical staff who check in specimens, enter data, and undertake the normal office work of the department. There are also the laboratory technicians who are highly skilled in the laboratory methods used with different specimens and micro-organisms. There are also medical staff who, with the help of the technical staff, interpret results and advise other clinicians on appropriate therapy.

Thus the laboratory personnel are not only involved in the handling of specimens (Shanson, 1991), but also contribute to:

- the diagnosis of the infection;
- identifying the causative organism;
- advice on the correct antibiotic regimes;
- the early detection of clusters of infection and antibiotic resistance.

These activities are achieved in a variety of ways.

- Microbiological examination of specimens. The laboratory is organised to ensure that the relevant tests are undertaken according to the specimen and the information available.
- Liaison with other HCWs. In the hospital microbiology laboratory, staff communicate with clinicians and will visit patients on wards. In the community the same discussions occur between GPs and microbiologists. In addition there is liaison with the Consultant in Communicable Disease Control and Environmental Health Officers.
- Infection control. In the hospital the medical microbiologist is normally

appointed as the Infection Control Doctor (ICD). Policies on the use of antibiotics, infection control precautions, isolation procedures and decontamination are drawn up by the hospital infection control committee which includes the ICD. The ICD, with the Infection Control Nurse will also investigate any evidence of cross-infection.

- Education and research. All medical, nursing and pharmacy staff need to receive education on the use of antibiotics and disinfectants. Any HCW who is involved in the collection and handling of specimens should also receive some education in the methods used and they must also be aware of safety regulations. Written information should also be available. Special precautions for the handling of 'high risk' specimens must be defined by the laboratory and the hospital management.

Research may consist of looking at new diagnostic techniques in the laboratory, the effectiveness of treatment regimens, or epidemiological research. In addition, the network of laboratories who are part of the public health laboratory service (PHLS) provide services for testing water, food and milk supplies. The PHLS laboratories also assist the hospital laboratories in the investigation of outbreaks of infection in the hospital and community and provide valuable information in the form of published research and epidemiological papers. The central public health laboratory based in Colindale, North London produces weekly communicable disease reports for England and Wales. This ensures that data are collected and looked at on a countrywide level. However, for historical and legal reasons, in the UK, England and Wales, Scotland and Northern Ireland all have separate reporting requirements and systems.

METHODS USED IN THE LABORATORY

Transport of specimens

Many microbes can perish on the way to the laboratory. To overcome the frequent inevitable delay in specimens reaching the laboratory the following methods may be used:

- transport media, such as Stuart's medium;
- boric acid, which may be added to urine;
- dip slide, for inoculating urine in clinics;
- refrigeration, storage at 4°C before processing will prevent the multiplication of most bacteria;
- freezing, temperatures of −7°C or below will preserve many microbes.

The microbiology laboratory aims to reproduce the conditions in which pathogenic micro-organisms grow so that the causative organism can be identified. Types of specimens received by the laboratory include:

- urine;
- blood;
- faeces;
- sputum;
- wound swabs;
- aspirated specimens;
- tissue biopsy.

The microbiology laboratory requires enough information on the request form to use the best methods to identify potential pathogens and this is why it is so important that all areas of the form are completed, not just where the specimen is from but relevant medical history and travel abroad. The specimen must also be collected with care to prevent contamination with commensals or other external sources and it is essential to use sterile containers which are leakproof and able to withstand transportation through the post if necessary. The specimens must then be transported to the laboratory quickly in the appropriate manner.

Microscopy and culture

Microscopy

A standard light microscope is the most common piece of equipment used, although other techniques such as immunofluorescence and electron microscopy are available. The electron microscope enables very small objects to be visualised, e.g. 0.0001μm.

Prior to microscopy the specimen has to be prepared. Slide films are divided into stained, unstained or wet film.

- Stained film. Christian Gram developed a quick and easy method of colouring cells with dyes in 1884 and this is still the most frequently used method (Sleigh and Timbury, 1990). Other methods include staining for acid fast bacilli (AFB) and alcohol fast bacilli, e.g. tubercle bacilli. Other special stains are used to help demonstrate capsules, spores and flagella.
- Unstained or wet film. Drops of liquid specimen or fluid culture are placed on a slide and covered with a cover slip. This method can show bacteria and cells as well as the movement of bacteria.

Microscopy and Gram staining are investigations which can be undertaken quickly and often provide a provisional identification if the infection is life-threatening.

Culture

It is important to ensure that bacteria do not die *en route* to the laboratory; for this reason transport medium is used. Culture of the specimen shows the growth of bacteria following incubation at a controlled temperature in the laboratory, designed to ensure optimal growth.

Bacteria grow well on artificial media. However, as different bacteria have different growth requirements many different media are needed. The majority of bacteria grow on blood agar. Media may be solid or liquid (for blood cultures a greater surface area is achieved with a liquid medium. It is also obviously impractical to pour blood onto a solid agar plate).

The bacteria are incubated at around body temperature, and it normally takes 24 hours until there are enough bacteria present for further testing. Some specimens are incubated in an oxygen-free environment if it is thought that the pathogens may be anaerobes.

Constituents of culture medium
Culture medium consists of:

- water;
- sodium chloride;
- peptone; a protein, animal or vegetable;
- meat extract;
- yeast extract;
- blood, usually horse;
- agar, carbohydrate derived from seaweed.

It is usually supplied commercially in a dehydrated form, reconstituted and sterilized in the laboratory before use.

Media for blood culture
This is contained in two bottles with rubber caps. The blood is collected using an aseptic procedure and is inoculated into the bottles. One contains nutrients for aerobic culture and the second nutrients for anaerobic culture

Identifying the bacteria

The culturing methods allow growth of any bacteria present in the specimen. Initially an experienced laboratory worker may be able to identify bacteria from the appearance of the colonies, which can be seen on the agar plates with the naked eye. The conditions in which the bacteria have grown will also aid this initial identification.

Most laboratories use commercially prepared kits for further identification tests (Sleigh and Timbury, 1990). These tests are prepared so that the chemical changes which take place after the specimen has been inoculated onto the test medium and then incubated, allow for the accurate identification of a particular bacteria. Some bacteria, e.g. *Staphylococcus aureus*, are identified by the production of a characteristic enzyme. Immunological techniques are also used. This serological method is considered the most reliable as these methods recognise the particular antigen which is specific to a particular bacterial species.

It is often necessary to identify individual strains or types within a particular bacterial species and this is termed typing. There are three main methods of typing:

- antigenic;
- bacteriophage;
- bacteriocine.

The importance of typing is that there are often many different strains of each bacterial species and during the investigation of cross-infection and outbreaks it is essential to be able to be as specific about the bacteria as possible. Typing is fairly expensive, and not all laboratories have this facility. However, the network of public health reference laboratories accept specimens for typing, and feed the results back to the requesting laboratory.

Antibiotic sensitivity tests

These tests form the bulk of the laboratory workload and provide vital information for the microbiologists when advising on antimicrobial treatment of patients. Two main methods are used.

Disc diffusion
These are paper discs impregnated with antibiotic solutions which are placed on the surface of the agar plate and then inoculated all over with the specimen or bacterial culture. When there is growth of the bacteria right up to the disc, it is said that the bacteria is resistant to that particular antibiotic at that concentration. The antibiotic concentrations used on the discs are the same as those that would be found by testing blood or urine of a patient receiving the antibiotic.

Tube dilution
This is only undertaken in special circumstances when there are concerns over difficulties in antibiotic treatment. A series of tubes each containing double doses of antibiotic from the previous one are inoculated with bacteria. The tube which contains the lowest dose of antibiotic to inhibit bacterial growth indicates the minimum inhibitory concentration (MIC) of the antibiotic required to prevent growth.

The laboratory also provides facilities to test specimens from patients on antibiotic treatment to ensure that:

- the concentration of the antibiotic in the blood is below a level associated with severe side effects e.g. toxicity;
- the concentration of the antibiotic in the blood is adequate to eliminate the bacteria.

In these cases blood specimens are taken before and after the antibiotic is administered. Regimens can then be adjusted dependent on the results.

Serology

Some diseases are still diagnosed by looking for the antibodies that the body produces to a specific bacteria. The results are expressed as a titre.

Identification of viruses

Unlike bacteria, viruses do not grow on artificial media. They can only grow on living cells. To achieve this, living cells are grown on nutrient medium on glass or plastic in the virology department. When grown in the laboratory, viruses alter the living cells upon which they are growing on in certain ways, enabling identification. However, not all viruses will grow on tissue culture. Some need to be stained by using special techniques. Viruses are also identified using electron microscopy.

Serological tests

As with some diseases caused by bacteria, viral illnesses may be detected by the appearance of antibodies to the specific virus in the patient's blood. This process is used extensively to diagnose viral infections. The most commonly used method is the enzyme linked immunosorbent assay (ELISA) test (Timbury, 1994). To achieve this an antigen specific to the antibody to be detected is incubated with serum from the patient. A colour change indicates the reaction.

Serum antibodies

During the course of an infection, different antibodies can be detected in the blood. These show whether someone has had the infection in the past or is still recovering from the infection. In the case of the virus hepatitis B, the different types of antibody present also show if the patient is a carrier of the disease.

THE COLLECTION AND PROCESSING OF SPECIMENS FOR LABORATORY EXAMINATION

In the past it was generally accepted that requesting specimens and laboratory investigations was a medical responsibility, and that the nursing responsibility lay only in collecting the specimens. However, more and more nurses are initiating specimen taking nowadays, particularly in areas such as midwifery where nurses are educated to a high degree and feel competent to undertake many tasks which 20 years ago were seen as the responsibility of the medical staff. To ensure that specimens are being requested for the right reasons and that request forms are being completed correctly, nurses and midwives need to be trained in these areas as well as the more traditional area of specimen collection. Incomplete or incorrect request forms with poor clinical information may result in inadequate, misleading or delayed laboratory reports (Ayliffe *et al.*, 1992), thus affecting patient care.

Request forms

Routine clinical information that should be stated on request forms includes the following:

- age of patient;
- relevant clinical information;
- date of onset of symptoms;
- recent or current antibiotic treatment;
- antibiotic allergies if known;
- history of recent travel abroad;
- nature of specimen, e.g. urine, catheter sample or mid-stream urine;
- specific anatomical site of wound swab;
- additional information such as employment, contact with others who have similar symptoms.

Specimen collection

It is vital that the correct specimen is collected using a method that will produce a usable specimen. Also, it is essential that further infection of the patient is prevented and that the infection risk to the person collecting the specimen is minimised through using universal infection control precautions (UICP).

Risk to staff

The collection, transportation and examination of biological specimens do pose a risk to staff. Extensive guidelines have been produced to provide precautions to protect workers and the environment (Advisory Committee on Dangerous Pathogens, 1995; Health Services Advisory Committee, 1992).

Prevention of contamination

To prevent the possibility of contamination the following points should always be followed:

- specimen bags should be sealed correctly;
- the specimen request form should be in a separate compartment from the specimen;
- if the request form becomes contaminated another form should be completed;
- the outside of the specimen container must not be contaminated.

Transporting specimens

Specimens should be transported from hospital wards/clinics, operating departments, GP practices, nursing homes etc. in strong leak-proof boxes made of non-porous easy-to-clean material. The health services advisory committee recommends autoclaving these boxes once a week.

Postal transportation

If specimens are posted, details of packaging and labelling requirements are set out by the Post Office in a document entitled *Inland Postal Services Prohibitions*. A copy of this can be obtained by contacting any main post office.

Practical aspects of safe and effective specimen collection and transportation

All specimens should be regarded as potentially infectious and all HCWs should follow universal infection control precautions when collecting and handling specimens. In most instances staff will need to wear protective clothing in the form of clean gloves when taking specimens.

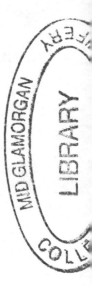

Swabs

Swabs may be collected from the throat, wounds or vagina. During collection it is important to avoid contamination of the container rim with the infected material or swab. Any spatula used during the collection process must be discarded as clinical waste. If pus is present this should be collected and sent in preference to a swab. Swabs should be placed in a transport medium, for example Stuart's Medium, to preserve the bacteria on its journey to the laboratory.

Special swab kits are available to diagnose whooping cough (pertussis), and where chlamydial infection is suspected. Swabs for viral culture require a special viral transport medium, which normally needs to be kept under refrigeration.

Faecal specimens

These may be sent to detect bacteria, viruses, ova, cysts and parasites. More than one specimen may be required as the causative organism is not always found during the first investigation. Only a small amount of faeces or faecal fluid need be sent. Faecal specimens on rectal swabs are usually unsuitable (Ayliffe et al., 1992).

Urine specimens

Urine in the bladder is normally sterile. However, it is very easy to contaminate specimens through poor collection techniques. This can lead to an inaccurate diagnosis in the laboratory, or in the case of catheter specimens may actually introduce infection during collection.

Ideally, specimens should be examined within two hours of collection. If this is not possible, the specimen should be refrigerated at 4°C to prevent bacterial growth. When transport to the laboratory is difficult and specimens cannot be examined for up to 24 hours then boric acid can be used in the containers to prevent bacterial growth. Three types of urine specimens are collected:

- mid-stream specimen of urine (MSU);
- clean catch specimen;
- catheter specimen of urine (CSU).

Collection of urine specimens

Mid-stream specimen

- Clean genital area prior to collecting.
- Discard the first flow of urine.
- Collect mid-flow in sterile universal container.
- Empty rest of bladder into toilet/commode.

Clean catch specimen This is collected when bladder control is poor.

- Clean the genital area.
- Collect the flow of urine in a universal container (as above).

Catheter specimen of urine This is collected from the sampling sleeve of the urinary drainage system. It is an aseptic procedure using a sterile syringe and fine bore needle.

Aspirated fluids

Fluids may be aspirated from the thoracic cavity, joints, facial sinuses and cerebrospinal spaces. It is a sterile procedure to avoid contamination of the specimen.

Sputum specimens

These should be obtained in a sterile container. HCWs should wear gloves when collecting these specimens. To protect porters and laboratory staff the rim of the container should be wiped to remove any contamination which may occur during collection. The tissue should be discarded as clinical waste. Three specimens are required for suspected cases of tuberculosis.

Blood specimens

When finger-prick specimens are taken, individual single-use devices are essential and should be disposed of immediately after use into a sharps container. Devices are now available whereby the sharp retracts after use, thus making this procedure and disposal of the used device less hazardous. Blood cultures when taken must be transferred to an incubator immediately. Blood culture bottles have expiry dates and these should be checked. The specimen should be taken directly from a vein, not an intravenous device, the skin should be disinfected before use and care taken not to contaminate the needle or blood culture bottle top.

Biopsy materials

Biopsy material is transported upright in either Ringers solution or sterile saline. If microbiological examination is required then formalin or fixatives should not be used.

Transport media and processing

Microbiological swabs

Microbiological specimens contain transport media, which is a bacterial culture enabling organisms to survive but not to increase in numbers. Taking a swab is an inexact science; it is possible to obtain a swab which contains a disproportionate amount of one particular type of organism. This is why it is important that if a wound is being swabbed because it is believed to be infected that the swab is taken as near as possible to the infected, red and inflamed area as possible. If pus is present it is better to send this than a wound swab.

Viral culture

Viral transport medium contains antibiotics. Different media contain different antibiotics depending on the type of organism suspected of causing the infection. Viruses cannot grow in the medium itself as it does not contain living cells.

Time delay

If any delay is suspected the swab should be stored in the refrigerator. However, it should be noted that, if this is done, the numbers will be depleted, and meningococcus and gonococcus will die.

Amount

It is only necessary to send a small amount of urine and stool.

Laboratory reports

Once the results of specimens are known, it is vital that this information is passed on to the relevant person quickly (Greenwood *et al.*, 1992). Generally, information is given on a laboratory report form. However, when results need to be communicated urgently, telephones and faxes are often used.

REFERENCES

Advisory Committee on Dangerous Pathogens (1995) *Categorisation of Biological Agents According to the Hazard and Categories of Containment*, 4th edn, HMSO, London.

Ayliffe, G.A.J., Lowbury, E.J.L. *et al.* (1992) *Control of Hospital Infection. A practical handbook*, 3rd ed, Chapman & Hall Medical, London .

Greenwood, D., Slack, R. and Peutherer, J. (1992) *Medical Microbiology. A Guide to Microbial Infections: Pathogenesis, Immunity, Laboratory Diagnosis and Control*, 14th ed, Churchill Livingstone, London.

Health Services Advisory Committee (1992) *Safe Working and Prevention of Infection in Clinical Laboratories – Model Rules for Staff and Visitors*, HMSO, London.

Shanson, D. (1991) *Microbiology in Clinical Practice*, 2nd ed, Butterworth and Company Publication Ltd, London, UK.

Sleigh, J.D. and Timbury, M. (1990) *Medical Microbiology*, 3rd ed, Churchill Livingstone, London.

Timbury, M.C. (1994) *Notes on Medical Virology*, 10th ed, Churchill Livingstone, London.

FURTHER READING

Advisory Committee on Dangerous Pathogens (1990) *HIV – the Causative Agent of AIDS and Related Conditions*, 2nd revision of guidelines, HMSO, London.

Advisory Committee on Dangerous Pathogens (1990) *Categorization of Pathogens According to Hazard and Categories of Containment*, 2nd edn, HMSO, London.

Advisory Task Force on Standards to the Audit Steering Committee of the Royal College of Pathologists (1991) Pathology departments accreditation in the United Kingdom: a synopsis. *Journal of Clinical Pathology*, **44**, 798–802.

Caddow, P. (ed.) (1990) *Applied Microbiology*, Scutari Press, London.

Cooke, E.M. (1991) *Hare's Bacteriology and Immunity for Nurses*, 7th ed, Churchill Livingstone, London.

Mandell, G.L., Douglas, R.G. and Bennett, J.E. (eds) (1994) *Principles and Practice of Infectious Diseases*. 4th ed., Churchill Livingstone, London.

Meers, P., Sedgwick, J., McPherson, M. (1997) *Infection Control in Healthcare*, Stanley Thornes, Cheltenham.

Stucke, V. (1993) *Microbiology for Nurses: Applications to Patient Care*, 7th ed, Baillière Tindall, London.

Worsley, M., Ward, K., Parker, L., et al. (eds) (1990) *Infection Control Guidelines for Nursing Care*, ICNA, London.

3 | The UK Health Service

The National Health Service has seen many changes and reorganisations in the past 20 years, but many health care staff remain unclear why the most recent changes occurred, or how they affect their role. This brief history and overview of today's NHS is intended to place the function of infection control in the overall context.

THE HISTORY OF THE NHS

The notion of a comprehensive and universal national health care system in the UK was first conceived during the Second World War, and was implemented by the post-war Labour government on 5th July 1948. The coalition had initially considered a decentralised and pluralistic system based upon voluntary and municipal hospitals. However this was significantly amended by the incoming Labour health secretary Aneurin Bevan who wished to see a more centralised and unitary system, with a nationalised hospital sector. The health service structure in the late 1990s more closely resembles the original Beveridge Report of 1942 in this respect.

The service structure changed little during the 50s and 60s, with both the Labour and Conservative parties recognising that the NHS needed to develop a more strategic capacity to counter the service's apparent loss of direction.

1974 reorganisation

In 1974 the service was reorganised creating 14 Regional Health Authorities (RHAs) in England with responsibility for planning, building and finance. In addition, 19 new Area Health Authorities (AHAs) were created below them with responsibility for family practitioner services, managed by Family Practitioner Committees (FPCs), which included general practitioners, dentists, pharmacists and opticians. Community health care services which had previously been managed by local government were also transferred to the responsibility of the NHS by the 1974 reforms. The arrangements in Scotland, Wales and Northern Ireland were slightly different, reflecting the strategic capacity that already existed in the Civil Service. Community Health Councils (CHCs) were also created with the aim of introducing local accountability, although their function was only advisory.

This new strategic capacity tackled the development and implementation of a new formula for allocating funding within the NHS. Named after the Resource Allocation Working Party (RAWP) which developed it, funding was allocated on a range of variables, such as social deprivation, age and sex. As a consequence, regions, areas and local hospitals became known as RAWP gaining, losing or neutral, with the London region in particular being subjected to significant reductions in its allocation.

Although the NHS was more integrated than it had been in the past, many of the national policies or strategic initiatives struggled to get off the ground. Perhaps the bureaucracy of too many management tiers was partly responsible, but much of the power of the NHS remained in the hands of the medical profession, whose professional autonomy could be exercised to resist change very effectively.

The 1982 reorganisation

During the 1970s, concerns about underfunding regularly surfaced, and the increase of unionisation throughout the country, particularly among nurses and ancillary grades resulted in the 'winter of discontent' in 1978/79 when significant numbers of health service workers went on strike for the first time. The Royal Commission on the NHS had been established in 1976, but by the time it reported in July 1979 a new Conservative government had been elected and the incoming Thatcher government saw nothing of benefit in the report. The Black Report (Black, 1980), which was published in April 1979, advocated an integrated programme involving health services, employment, housing, etc. This was also largely ignored by the new Conservative administration. Of more significance was the consultative document *Patients First* (DHSS and Welsh Office, 1979) which suggested the removal of the area tier and the establishment of District Health Authorities (DHAs). This document suggested that patients would be better served if management decisions were made by people who had closer contact with the patient. It also recommended that the professional consultative machinery should be simplified, and that the hierarchy of functional management should be dismantled and be replaced by unit management teams, being typically responsible for a hospital or local community service.

Further reorganisation occurred in 1982. The Conservative government began changing the management culture and, faced with escalating health costs, proposed ways to encourage patients to use private hospitals and nursing homes. Health authorities were also required to put their support services, such as domestic, cleaning, laundry and catering out to competitive tender, allowing private firms to manage and run parts of the Health Service for the first time since 1948.

The introduction of general management

In 1983, dissatisfaction with the consensus style of management began to grow, with critics complaining that managing by mutual consent allowed professions, and in particular doctors, to procrastinate over proposed changes. The Secretary of State responded by establishing a team of four businessmen led by Roy Griffiths, the then managing director of Sainsbury's, to advise him. The Griffiths' Report (Griffiths, 1983) was published in October 1983 as the NHS Management Inquiry.

The Griffiths' Report identified the lack of accountability within the service, and advised that general managers should be appointed at all levels within the service to drive through the improvements and increase the efficiency of the organisation. It also suggested that the Secretary of State should establish and chair a health service supervisory board, with a management board accountable to it. Joining the Secretary of State would be the Minister of State (Health), the Permanent Secretary of the Department of Health and Social Security, the Chief Medical Officer and the Chairman of the Management Board. The idea was that the management board would be the executive arm of the supervisory board, implementing national policies and giving leadership to the management of the service.

Professional autonomy

The White Paper *Working for Patients* (DoH, 1989) was published in January 1989, probably in response to the increasing financial demands on the service. There was also a mixture of pragmatism and an ideological dogma based on the belief that a private sector business culture could provide better quality public services more efficiently. The government also suspected that doctors and managers both had vested interests in influencing public opinion to demand more and more resources for the NHS managers, distracting them from attacking the inefficiencies and clinicians' resistance to change. Efficiency scrutinies and performance indicators, although crude, indicated significant differences in lengths of stay and cost per case between hospitals. Although cost reductions and improvements had been made since 1982, it was recognised that performance-related pay for many senior managers would leave unchallenged the presumption of professional autonomy. The White Paper provoked considerable criticism, particularly from professionals, but the Bill received Royal Consent as the National Health Service and Community Care Act on 29th June 1990.

The new legislation replaced the supervisory board with a policy board, and the NHS Management Executive, led by a chief executive, was accountable to it. Health authorities which until this time had been made up of between 15 and 20 members representing a broad range of political and professional interests, were replaced by something closer in style to the commercial world, with executive and non-executive components held in balance by a 'chair'.

NHS trusts

The change in health authority structure was a fundamental cultural change for the NHS. However, even this issue was overshadowed by the debate about establishing NHS trusts which, released from the bureaucracy of DHA management, would be free to operate their own 'market' for patient care, and be able to pay staff outside national agreements. The trusts were to be established with their own management boards and could raise money more freely. The establishment of trusts was seen by many as the privatisation of the NHS, despite the government's insistence that health care would continue to be provided free at the point of delivery, and would be financed mainly from taxation.

In December 1990, 56 hospital and community care trusts were established, while those management units that remained under the control of the DHA were known as directly-managed units. However, by 1996, virtually all hospital and community care units in the UK were trusts.

Trust boards are composed of a chairman, and a balance of executive and non-executive directors, totalling a maximum of 11, including the chairman. The chairman is appointed by the Secretary of State, with two of the non-executive directors appointed by the RHAs. Following the dissolution of RHAs this responsibility falls to the Secretary of State. If a trust is associated with a university, and provides a teaching function, then the dean or other university official is appointed as a director.

The choice of executive directors is rather more prescriptive, and must include the chief executive, the director of finance, a medical practitioner, and a registered nurse or registered midwife. (Obviously there are exceptions for trust boards responsible for functions such as an ambulance service.) The chairman and all board non-executives need to be re-appointed after four years, although executive directors are permitted to hold their offices for the period of their trust employment.

Contracting

Although NHS trusts had greater financial freedoms, in many ways directly managed units were treated in the same way by DHAs who were charged with purchasing health care for the local population. DHAs were funded on the basis of their resident population, and were required to pay for the treatment of patients whether it be provided by provider units. Previously, DHA allocations had been based upon historical referral patterns; for example patients who travelled up to London from Exeter for treatment were, in effect, funded by the London health authority rather than the health authority of residence. From 1991, financial agreements or contracts were devised between health authorities and the provider units. For the first time, DHAs could begin to influence where a patient was treated, and local hospital and community providers could no longer guarantee that their historical referral patterns would continue. This introduced a form of market competition between health care providers, and encouraged some health authorities to put a few clinical services out for competitive tender, with the purpose of achieving the best quality and value for money for their local residents.

DHAs began to insist that as many patients as possible should be treated locally where appropriate health services existed, rather than allowing a patient to travel to a large teaching hospital centred in, for example, Birmingham, Bristol, Leeds or London. The more specialist procedures that many of these institutions offer still continued to attract patients from all round the country, but financial authorisation for the treatment often needed to be sorted out in advance before it could commence. Emergencies are not subject to this requirement of prior authorisation, but, where a contract is not in place, hospitals will invoice districts on an individual patient basis after treatment.

The majority of patients are, of course, treated at their local hospital under block contracts, and this removes the need for individual patient billing. Nevertheless criticism has built over recent years that the purchaser–provider split between health authority and trust has increased bureaucracy.

GP fundholders

Although DHAs were responsible for the bulk of NHS spending for their local residents, some general practitioners were given the opportunity to hold budgets for a range of treatments (mainly elective surgical procedures). Practices that became 'fund holders' gained greater influence over hospital provision and have altered the relative balance of power between general practice and hospital medicine. Early on in their introduction, some observers were concerned that a two-tier service was beginning to develop between fund holding and non-fundholding GPs.

In April 1996, the sixth wave of GP fundholders was introduced, and it is estimated that over 50% of the population are covered by GP fundholders. Many have formed partnerships (sometimes referred to as multifunds) and their combined purchasing power may exceed that of their local health authority.

Purchasers and providers

The separation of purchasing and providing has undoubtedly improved the responsiveness of providers to patient's needs and has improved services. The influence of GP fundholders has acted as a catalyst to improve the quality of service delivery, as they have insisted on improved waiting times and better continuity of care between the hospital and general practitioners. The split has also permitted health authorities to focus on the difficult task of assessing the health needs of their local population, and to pursue the development of primary and community care services which, it is often claimed, have lost out in the allocation of resources to the previously dominant acute services.

Considerable effort is being spent to ensure that performance of the trusts can be measured and compared on a similar basis, and teaching hospitals and special health authorities are working to identify separately the teaching and research costs currently integrated into the overall cost of the service.

However the implementation of the White Paper continues to evolve, with some fundholders now piloting the purchasing of all health care to meet their patient's needs, that is to say both emergency and elective care.

Special health authorities

The NHS reforms also presented an opportunity for special health authorities (e.g. the Royal Marsden and Brompton hospitals), which had previously been excluded from the traditional NHS funding system to be brought into the fold, and became subject to NHS contracts and market pressures in the same way as other NHS providers.

Family health service authorities (FHSAs)

FHSAs were established following the abolition of AHAs, replacing the FPCs. Until recently they have remained independent from DHAs.

However, in 1995, the Health Authorities Act was passed, permitting the integration of FHSAs and DHAs, within one single authority now responsible for both acute, primary and community care for its local residents.

Continuing care and *The Health of the Nation*

The second White Paper published in 1989 was intended to sort out the responsibility for patients requiring continuing care, especially the elderly and people with learning or physical disabilities. While local authorities had the responsibility of providing social care, health care was provided by the NHS. However the overlap in the provision of these services caused confusion, and under the NHS and Community Care Act 1990, the local authorities were given the responsibility as the lead agency in the provision of community care, contracting with the NHS and other agencies to ensure that a proper care plan is formulated and implemented for each patient.

With the increase in opportunities for patients to receive care in private and charitable sectors, the powers of the social services inspectorate were increased to maintain standards and good practice. In addition, because there was to be an individual budget for each assessed person, the method of income support was reformed. *Caring for People* (DHSS, 1989), which was the government's response to the community care proposals made by Griffiths, was introduced slowly, as the cost of intro-

Table 3.1 Summary of key changes in the NHS structure, and important Acts of Parliament

NHS established	1948
Management arrangements for the reorganised NHS	1974
Management reorganisation	1982
Griffiths' Report	1983
Mental Health Act	1983
Registered Homes Act	1984
Resource Management Initiative	1986
Working for Patients	1989
Caring for People	1989
Children Act	1989
NHS and Community Care Act	1990
Patient's Charter	1991
Health of the Nation	1992
Managing the new NHS	1993
Health Authorities Act	1995

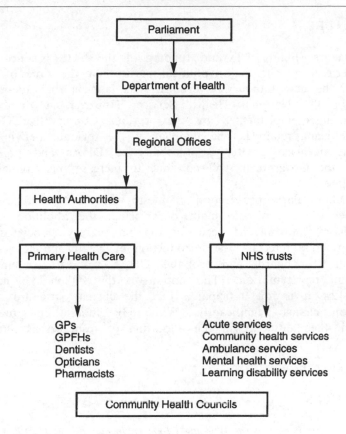

Figure 3.1 The structure of the National Health Service

ducing the poll tax or community charge coincided with the requirement for local health authorities to cope with the financial burden of introducing new methods of supporting dependent people in the community as well.

The third White Paper, the *Health of the Nation* (DoH, 1992) was published in July 1992, with the aim of providing a new national strategy focused on health rather than health care. Targets were set in the areas of coronary heart disease, cancers, mental illness, HIV/AIDS, sexual health and accidents. The White Paper represented a significant recognition of the role of preventative medicine and health promotion, emphasising the need for multi-disciplinary and intersectoral approaches between government departments, local authorities, the independent sector and the individuals themselves. A summary of the key changes in NHS structure and important Acts of Parliament is shown in Table 3.1.

THE FUTURE

The structure (Figure 3.1) and funding of the NHS is once again being debated by the major political parties. At the time of going to press, the new Labour Government has launched a wide-ranging review of the National Health Service. However, a number of recent changes implemented by the previous Conservative Government are being retained. The removal of the regional tier in April 1996 has devolved greater responsibility to DHAs and providers, although the Government will continue to increase measurements of performance.

The Labour Party pre-election manifestos on the NHS focused on a number of themes, the main ones being: the abolition of the marketplace, removing the need for the bureaucracy associated with extra-contractual referrals; the introduction of greater public accountability on trust boards and probably DHAs, with greater emphasis on patient representation. (The notion of the stakeholder nation.) Nevertheless, it is not anticipated that the current structure of the NHS will change significantly. While GP fundholding may be abolished, their influence in the allocation of resources is likely to remain.

REFERENCES

Black, D. (1980) *Report of the Working Group on Inequalities in Health*, HMSO, London.

Dept. of Health (1989) *Working for Patients. The Health Service Caring for the 1990s*, CM555, HMSO, London.

Dept. of Health (1992) *The Health of the Nation. A Strategy for Health in England*, HMSO, London.

DHSS (1989) *Caring for People: Community Care in the Next Decade and Beyond*, CM849, HMSO, London.

DHSS and Welsh Office (1979) *Patients First*, HMSO, London.

Griffiths, R. (1983) Report of NHS Management Inquiry. Published under cover of a letter from Sir Roy Griffiths to the Secretary of State for Social Services, 6th October 1983. Chairman Sir Roy Griffiths. *Tech. Rep.*

FURTHER READING

Adler, J. and Tofts, A. (1996) Croner's *Health Service Manager*, Croner Publications Ltd, Kingston-upon-Thames.

Holliday, I. (1995) *The NHS Transformed*, 2nd ed, Baseline Book Company, Manchester.

Levitt, R., Wall, A. and Appleby, J. (1995) *The Reorganised National Health Service*, 5th ed, Chapman & Hall, London.

NHS Executive (1996) *A Guide to the National Health Service*, NHS Executive Communications Unit, London.

Structure and function of infection control

As the twentieth century draws to a close and we enter into the twenty-first, the nature and distribution of communicable diseases and infection continues to present a challenge to health care professionals. Diseases that were thought to be no longer a problem in the 1970s and early 1980s, e.g. tuberculosis are again causing concern. New blood borne viruses are being discovered, such as HIV, and hepatitis viruses. Outbreaks of infection occur frequently and the number of reported cases of food poisoning from *Salmonella* spp. and *Campylobacter* spp. are increasing. Medical care is becoming increasingly complex, which has an affect on hospital acquired infection (HAI). The emergence of multi-drug resistant organisms, ever more invasive techniques and the need to cut health care costs has shown the importance of accurate research-based infection control advice.

In the general population, infection control is practised through the provision of adequate fresh food and water and by satisfactory waste disposal including sewage and refuse. The huge improvement in medical knowledge and easy access to medical care has made the UK population healthier and has increased life expectancy. This increased life expectancy has brought its own problems with more and more of the population in the UK aged over 65 years, having chronic diseases which require care, and which can make the individual more susceptible to infection.

THE FUNCTION OF INFECTION CONTROL

Hospital

Hospital infection control is an important part of an effective risk management programme. The Control of Substances Hazardous to Health Regulations (COSHH), 1994, includes pathogenic micro-organisms among the hazards. Other health and safety at work legislation and food legislation imposes obligations on hospitals. Ethically, hospitals are obliged to prevent avoidable infections in their patients and, with more people in the UK becoming aware of their rights under the patient's charter, those who become infected are increasingly likely to take legal action against a hospital that they believe to have been negligent.

Infection control in UK hospitals functions in the following way. The responsibility for ensuring that there are effective arrangements for infection control rests with the trust's chief executive. In the UK most hospitals have an infection control team (ICT), and a hospital infection control committee (HICC). The ICT has the primary responsibility for the surveillance, prevention and control of infection in the hospital. The ICT comprises the infection control doctor (ICD), the infection control nurse(s) (ICNs) and a hospital manager. The ICD reports directly to the chief executive on all matters related to infection control.

The ICD is normally a medical microbiologist, and should have a specialist interest in infection control. The ICN is usually the only full time member of the ICT, and has a specialist knowledge of infection control. The ICT provides advice on all matters related to infection control to all employees in the provider unit in which they work. The hospital manager gives advice and managerial support to decisions taken by the ICD and ICN. Full details of the roles of the ICD and ICN are given in Chapter 5.

The HICC is the organisation that regulates all infection control activities in the hospital. The two major roles of the committee are to translate the professional input of the ICT into formal policy ratified by the trust, and to disseminate infection control information to all clinical areas of the hospital. Full details of the various infection control committees are given in Chapter 6.

The community

Arrangements for the surveillance, prevention, treatment and control of communicable disease in a health district is one function of the public health department. The responsibility lies with the consultant in communicable disease control (CCDC) to make provision for, and co-ordinate infection control programmes in the health authority, the local authority and the community. Many CsCDC now have nurses experienced in infection control working with them.

INFECTION CONTROL SERVICE IN THE HOSPITAL

Guidance on infection control in the hospital is available in *Hospital Infection Control* (DHSS, 1995). The hospital must have adequate resources and arrangements for infection control, which will include infection control policies, and surveillance and training programmes. Hospital acquired infection (HAI) remains an important problem. The first national prevalence survey (Meers *et al.*, 1981) in England and Wales showed that 9.2% of patients surveyed had acquired an infection during their hospital stay. The results of a second UK wide survey conducted in 1993 and 1994, involving many more patients shows a prevalence rate of 9.0% (Emmerson *et al.*, 1996).

The cost of HAI is difficult to measure, as it is not just the extra days that patients spend in hospital or the cost of drugs, but must include, among other things, social and economic costs to the patient, loss of earnings and increased payments for childcare. Costs have been attempted worldwide which range from £21 to £3 010 per patient (DoH/PHLS, 1995). Most of these costs only include inpatient care. Indeed, if fresh water, sewage, laundry, food hygiene and waste disposal were all put under the umbrella of infection control it could be argued that at least one third of the total health care cost in the UK is as a result of infection control and prevention. However it is quantified, infection control does cost a lot of money, and it could be argued that more money should be put into the prevention component rather than the control.

Many health authorities are beginning to see infection rates as quality indicators and, throughout the UK, ICTs are beginning to take part in the surveillance of infections (Chapter 8). It has been estimated that in the 1990s about 30% of all HAI could be prevented by better application of existing knowledge and implementation of realistic infection control policies (DoH/PHLS, 1995).

Standards and audit

For the hospital infection teams to be able to audit the infection control practices in their provider units they need to have in place infection control standards. Agreed standards are available (IC Standards Working Party, 1993). Infection control standards should cover the following:

- structure and responsibilities in infection control;
- policies and procedures;
- surveillance;
- education.

Structure and responsibilities

Each provider unit should have an appropriate number of trained infection control practitioners with clearly defined responsibilities and level of accountability, and other resources to facilitate the prevention, detection and control of infection in the unit. This will include the following.

- An effective infection control committee (ICC) for each provider unit, with appropriate representation of other professional disciplines and management. This should meet a minimum of twice a year, and should prepare and review the annual infection control activities. The authority of the ICC, through its chairman, to institute any appropriate control measures or studies where there is reasonably considered to be a danger to any patient or health care worker, should be defined in writing and should be approved by the provider unit's chief executive.
- An infection control team (ICT) responsible for day to day infection control activity, with adequate support staff. The members of the ICT should be formally trained in infection control, and be regularly updated.
- Liaison with smaller units affiliated to the main unit, which may be through infection control link nurses (ICLNs).

Policies and procedures

The development of infection control guidelines should be initiated by the ICC and all members of the ICT and other staff in the provider unit should be involved in their development. The guidelines must be based on current legislation, and should be reviewed annually, and enforced as necessary.

- All guidelines which include references to infection control must have input from members of the ICC.
- All employees of the provider unit whether direct or contracted must be made aware of the appropriate infection control guidelines, either by attending induction programmes or update days.
- All guidelines should be audited regularly.

Surveillance

Surveillance of hospital acquired infection should be undertaken by the provider unit.

- There should be a written programme of surveillance, including priorities and definitions of nosocomial infections. All surveillance should be undertaken in collaboration with the provider unit's clinical staff.
- Effective measures should be in place to prevent, to identify and to control infections acquired in the hospital or brought into the hospital from the community.
- Data should be collected on a full time or part time basis by surveillance personnel who are qualified in such work. The data is analysed and the information is distributed to the relevant health care workers.
- There should be a practical system for reporting, evaluating and maintaining records of infections among patients.

Education

Resources are available for educational activities.

- There should be a budget for the ICT to attend conferences, study days and other relevant activities.
- The ICT has access to library resources.
- There is an educational programme relevant to different types of health care staff.

INFECTION CONTROL SERVICE IN THE COMMUNITY

Until 1974, the responsibility for the control of communicable disease rested entirely with the local authority, and was discharged by the Medical Officer of Health. This model had existed since 1871, and continued for 26 years after the founding of the NHS. However, in 1974, this local authority post was abolished and replaced by the post of 'community physician', which was a full time medical post in the NHS, thus dividing responsibility between the NHS and the local authority. These community physicians, who were also known as Medical Officers of Environmental Health (MOEH), were appointed as the proper officers for the Public Health Act. The separation of this function between the local authority and health authority has been a continued source of confusion. It was against this background that two major outbreaks of communicable disease – salmonella food poisoning at Stanley Royd Hospital in 1984 and legionnaires' disease in Stafford in 1985 – occurred, both of which resulted in public enquiries. The result of these enquiries was that a new post, that of the Consultant in Communicable Disease Control (CCDC) was created.

The role of the CCDC and community infection control nurse (CICN) is described in Chapter 5. The control of communicable disease requires a multidisciplinary approach. The expertise of local authority environmental health officers as regards the investigation of premises and food, water and other environmental vehicles of infection, is accepted as an essential component of the management of communicable disease. It is manifestly inseparable from their role as enforcers of food safety and other public health legislation.

It is equally clear that many of the communicable disease control activities, such as those to do with tuberculosis, meningitis, hepatitis B or HIV infection, can only be properly undertaken by medical or nursing personnel. These are addressed by immunisation, contact tracing or prophylactic treatment.

CsCDC are usually appointed as the proper officer by the local authority within their area. It is to the proper officer that notifiable diseases are reported (Chapter 8). It is also the proper officer who has the powers to constrain persons and control the environment.

The CCDC and CICN give infection control advice to many different types of people and establishments including trusts, general practices, dentists, schools, creches, nursing and residential homes, the local authorities and the private and voluntary sector within their area.

OCCUPATIONAL HEALTH

Occupational health has a vital role in infection control and members of the occupational health department work closely with the ICT in the hospital and liaise with the CCDC and CICN in the community. Occupational health staff have a specific role in that their work is centred on protecting individuals from the adverse effects of the environment. Health authorities, like all other employers in the UK have legal responsibilities to ensure that all their staff receive adequate training in how to prevent accidents and occupational diseases. While occupational health doctors and nurses and infection control practitioners may be specialists, other medical and nursing staff should be encouraged to co-operate in achieving a safe and healthy working environment.

Transmission of infection from patients to staff and vice versa in hospitals is well recognised (Ayliffe, 1992). Occupational health for hospital staff has been available since the late 1960s and, with the Health and Safety at Work Act (1974), most factories, large companies and hospitals have occupational health departments.

Risks to health care workers from patients/clients

By the very nature of the services they provide, hospitals are full of people who are ill and have infections and communicable diseases. Through giving care to patients HCWs put themselves at risk of acquiring infection. It is recognised that patients in hospital who have invasive procedures performed on them are more susceptible to infection. HCWs who perform these procedures are also at risk of acquiring infections, notably blood borne viruses. HCWs giving general care are at risk of acquiring infections occupationally, e.g. tuberculosis, HIV, hepatitis B and C and viral and bacterial gastrointestinal infections.

Staff have acquired blood borne viruses occupationally (Heptonstall *et al.*, 1993), and the risk of acquiring HIV became a major issue for HCWs and their employers in 1984 when the first case of a documented sero-conversion after percutaneous exposure to HIV infected blood at work was reported (Anon, 1984). This was one of the factors which enabled universal infection control precautions to be introduced (Chapter 9). The risk of acquiring, and then passing on hepatitis B virus is the reason behind the requirement for immunisation of all health care workers who undertake exposure prone procedures, e.g. surgeons and midwives (PHLS, 1992). Most provider unit occupational health departments will offer hepatitis B immunisation to all staff who may come into contact with blood or body fluid – this generally means most hospital staff. Staff who work in the community, e.g. in nursing and residential homes, sometimes have difficulty in obtaining hepatitis B immunisation from their general practitioner, and some have to pay. Employers should assess the risk of the procedures their employees perform and if they perceive a risk they should be offered hepatitis B immunisation, e.g. if there is a risk they may be bitten, or sustain a sharps injury.

Risks to patients from HCWs

The commonest infections in the community are the infections which are most frequently passed from HCWs to patients, e.g. colds, influenza, diarrhoea and vomiting. To stop these infections spreading in the hospital it is important that staff realise that coming to work with a cold, diarrhoea or vomiting puts their patients and their colleagues at risk. Unfortunately many staff will come to work when they are unwell, particularly if they are locum or agency staff and do not receive sick pay. It is vitally important that, all staff should be encouraged to co-operate in achieving a safe and healthy working environment. When a HCW may be a particular risk to their client group, such as if they are HIV positive or a hepatitis Be antigen carrier, the occupational health department has to advise staff on the safest course of action to be taken to reduce the risk of spread of infection to a reasonable level. This may mean that an HIV positive HCW can no longer practise in their chosen discipline. However it is important to remember that HIV positive and immunocompromised staff are also at risk from such diseases as multi-drug resistant tuberculosis.

Methicillin resistant *Staphylococcus aureus* (MRSA)

Staff have also been implicated in outbreaks of MRSA (Journal of Hospital Infection, 1990) and the question of staff screening has been raised. Often staff are screened when there is an outbreak, but even if they are found to be colonised with *Staphylococcus aureus* it might not be of the same strain or sensitivity as that causing the outbreak. The difficulty of staff screening is often overlooked. Frequently, only permanent hospital staff are screened; agency and locum staff are not. If staff are found to be positive the ICT and occupational health department are often unsure about the most appropriate course of action. These are questions that have to be answered prior to any screening being undertaken.

- If staff are sent off work, when can they return and what happens if MRSA carriage is not irradicated?
- Who will pay for an agency or locum member of staff to be put off work?

Pre-employment staff screening

All staff should be included in the initial screening and immunisation programme. This usually involves paper screening; the completion of a health questionnaire. If the answers are satisfactory the successful job applicant is employed. If there are any queries the applicant will be asked to attend the occupational health department before commencement of employment. Staff are also offered immunisation commensurate with the work they will undertake. All staff should be offered protection against tuberculosis, rubella and poliomyelitis. Laboratory and technical staff should be offered tetanus toxoid. Hepatitis B should be offered to anyone who may have contact with blood or body fluids.

REFERENCES

Anon (1984) Needlestick transmission of HTLV–111 from a patient infected in Africa. *Lancet*, **ii**, 1376–77.

Ayliffe, G.A.J., Lowbury, E.J.L., Geddes, A.M. and Williams, J.D. (1992) *Control of Hospital Infection. A practical handbook*, 3rd edn Chapman & Hall, London.

DHSS (1988) *Hospital Infection Control: General Management Arrangements*, HMSO, London.

DoH/PHLS (1995) Hospital Infection Working Group of the DoH and PHLS. Hospital Infection Control Guidance on the Control of Infection in Hospitals, HSG(95)10. *Tech. Rep.*

Emmerson, A.M., Enstone, J.E., Griffin, M. *et al.* (1996) The Second National Prevalence Survey of Infection in Hospitals – overview of the results. *Journal of Hospital Infection*, **32**, 175–90.

Heptonstall, J., Gill, O.N., Porter, K. *et al.* (1993) Health care workers and HIV: surveillance of occupationally acquired infection in the United Kingdom. *CDR Review*, **3** (11), R147–R153.

Journal of Hospital Infection (1990) Report of the combined working party of the hospital infection party and British Society of Antimicrobial Chemotherapy. Revised guidelines for the control of methicillin resistant *Staphylococcus aureus*. *Journal of Hospital Infection*, **16**, 351–770.

Meers, P.D., Ayliffe, G.A.J., Emmerson, A.M., *et al.* (1981) Report on the national survey of infection in hospitals. *Journal of Hospital Infection*, **2** (Supplement).

PHLS Hepatitis Subcommittee, (1992) Exposure to hepatitis B virus: guidance on post-exposure prophylaxis. *CDR Review*, **2**, (9), R97–101.

The Infection Control Standards Working Party (1993), *Standards in Infection Control in Hospitals*, HMSO, London

The infection control team | 5

The importance of controlling the spread of infection in hospital and the community has been recognised for a long time. In the latter half of the nineteenth century separate fever hospitals were built, although there was a certain amount of resistance from local residents (Abel-Smith, 1964). At the same time, smallpox victims were being cared for on ships borrowed from the Admiralty. By the early twentieth century there were 32 000 infectious diseases beds available (Abel-Smith, 1964). With the advent of antibiotics and immunisation the need for infectious diseases hospitals fell. However patients still acquire infections in the community and in hospitals, and it is the aim of the infection control practitioners to prevent, as far as possible, any infection from spreading from patient to patient, patient to staff or staff to patient.

The introduction of antibiotics in the 1940s, and their increasing availability in the late 1940s and 1950s led to the emergence of resistant *Staphylococcus aureus*. These 'hospital' staphylococci were the primary cause of hospital acquired infection. In 1944, hospitals in the UK were advised to set up infection control committees (ICCs) (Medical Research Council, 1944). Further recommendations followed (Ministry of Health, 1959), which led to hospitals appointing infection control officers (ICOs). In 1959, the first ICN in England was appointed in Torbay in Devon (Gardner, 1962). This was as a direct result of the difficulties that two Devon hospitals had had in controlling cross-infection. This first appointment proved highly successful (Prieto, 1994) and led to the appointment of more ICNs around the country.

In the USA, with the support of the Centers for Disease Control and Prevention in Atlanta, the surveillance and control of HAI was taken very seriously. Various professional bodies were established in Europe and the States and many articles and books have been written about infection control.

Every hospital should have an ICT (Chapter 4), and the roles of the hospital ICN and ICD are discussed below. As more CICNs are being appointed, their role is included here, together with the role of the consultant in communicable disease control (CCDC) both in the hospital and the community, and the role of the infection control link nurse (ICLN). A description of the role of the local authority environmental health officer is also given.

The prerequisite skills for the hospital ICD and ICN are a knowledge of hospital acquired infection, microbiology, virology, epidemiology, infectious diseases, and the workings of the provider unit. They must be able to communicate effectively with all grades of staff both verbally and on paper.

In the past, a job description for the ICN was always provided but there was rarely one for the ICD. With the recognition of the importance of infection control in the hospital setting, job descriptions for ICDs are now also available.

THE INFECTION CONTROL TEAM IN THE HOSPITAL

The infection control doctor (ICD)

Qualifications and experience

In the hospital, the ICD must be a registered medical practitioner formally trained in all aspects of infection control. The ICD is normally a consultant medical microbiologist, but in exceptional circumstances they may be an infectious diseases physician. A higher qualification is desirable, and this is usually membership of the Royal College of Pathologists (MRCPath).

The ICD should be trained in all aspects of infection and in the methods of its prevention and control, including epidemiology. It is essential that the ICD, through continuing education, remains up to date on all matters related to infection control, and there are regular educational training programmes available.

The ICD must be prepared to give a high priority to infection control and devote a substantial proportion of time to it. The job description should specify the average number of sessions per week that the ICD should devote to infection control, although there will be times, for example during outbreaks, when more time will be necessary.

Accountability

The ICD is appointed directly by the chief executive (CE) and will report direct to the CE.

Working relationships

The ICD works with:

- the infection control nurse(s);
- other consultant microbiologists;

- microbiology scientific staff;
- the chief executive;
- the trust board;
- the consultant(s) in communicable disease control;
- medical director;
- physicians;
- surgeons;
- occupational health department;
- other heads of department with infection control aspects of their work, e.g. catering, estates, pharmacy, CSSD, domestic services;
- outside bodies, e.g. public health laboratories, environmental health officers.

Overall responsibilities

The ICD will normally take the lead role in the effective functioning of the ICT. The ICT will include the infection control nurses (ICNs) and a consultant microbiologist if the ICD is from another specialty. The ICD attends all meetings and is an active member of the hospital infection control committee and, due to their acknowledged expertise, usually acts as chairperson. He/she, as part of the ICT, is one of the key people to draw up annual plans, policies, guidelines and procedures for the prevention of infection in the hospital setting. The ICD will also be an active member of the district infection control committee.

Some hospitals and trusts have more than one ICD. In these circumstances, the responsibilities of each must be clearly defined and their approaches must be agreed and consistent. One individual should take the lead on infection control matters, possibly on a rotating basis.

The role of the ICD

The ICD is responsible for a wide range of hospital infection control activities in the areas they cover, these include:

- Planning the infection control activity for the following year and writing the annual report with other members of the ICT.
- To serve as a specialist adviser, as outlined in joint DoH/PHLS guidelines on hospital infection control (1995), on all matters relating to hospital infection control. Such matters include surveillance and control aspects of hospital infection, sterilisation and disinfection methods, types of ventilation, operating theatres, isolation facilities, kitchens, laundries, housekeeping, waste disposal, pest control and antibiotic usage.
- To investigate outbreaks of hospital infection (Chapter 13). Close liaison with the consultant in communicable disease control (CCDC) is necessary.

- To prepare and update policies, together with other relevant personnel, in relation to hospital infection control, e.g. theatre polices, disinfection, sterilisation and patient isolation procedures.
- To co-ordinate the work of the ICT, which will include the ICN(s) and secretarial support.
- To act as chairperson or to be an active member of the hospital infection control committee.
- To advise the chief executive directly on all aspects of infection control in the hospital/trust and on implementation of agreed policies.
- To participate in the preparation of tender documents for support services, and advise on infection aspects of these services following award of a contract.
- To be involved in the setting of quality standards with regard to hospital infections, and in audits of infection.
- To be involved in the planning and upgrading of hospital facilities.
- To liaise with other ICDs and CsCDC in developing infection control programmes for the whole district.
- To take part in infection control training of all health care workers and students working in the hospital/trust.
- To advise and support the ICN in day to day activities.
- The ICD may delegate duties to other consultant colleagues, junior medical staff and the ICN.
- To make arrangements for the provision of infection control medical advice outside normal working hours.

Long stay and other non-acute and small hospitals, whether in the public or private sectors, will generally not have anyone among their medical staff who can fulfil the role of the ICD. They should therefore appoint an ICD who is based in a neighbouring acute hospital.

The infection control nurse

The first British infection control sister was appointed in 1959. Since then, the number of nurses employed full time in infection control in the UK, the USA and elsewhere in Europe has steadily grown. Most hospitals in the UK now have an ICN, however, there still remains some confusion about their status and their roles. Some ICNs view themselves as clinical nurse specialists, despite confusion over the meaning of the term (Prieto, 1994), which still requires clarification.

Qualifications and experience

The infection control nurse should be a registered nurse, with experience at ward manager level. For more senior posts, they should have the diploma in infection control or equivalent, and they should continue to keep up to date professionally once in post.

Accountability

The ICN is normally accountable to the ICD or the Director of Nursing.

Working relationships

The ICN works with:

- the infection control doctor (ICD);
- other infection control nurses;
- consultant microbiologists;
- staff of the microbiology laboratories;
- occupational health services;
- the consultant in communicable disease control (CCDC);
- educational establishments.

Overall responsibilities

The infection control nurse (together with the other members of the infection control team) is responsible for the management of surveillance and investigation of infections, and for advising on prevention and control measures within the provider unit.

The role of the ICN

The role of the ICN involves a variety of activities.

- To act as a specialist adviser to the executive of the provider unit and all employees in all matters relating to infection control.
- To advise and, if appropriate, assist in planning the care of individual patients with communicable infections.
- To inform staff on effective infection control standards.
- To investigate, with other members of the ICT, outbreaks of infection in the hospital environment to identify the source and mode of spread and advise on the appropriate infection control precautions to prevent further transmission.
- To advise on the disinfection, decontamination and cleaning of equipment.
- To provide expert advice to the supplies department on new equipment with reference to safe infection control practice and effective decontamination.
- The ICN is involved in planning, upgrading and capital projects within the trust.

- Participation in the preparation of tendering documents for support services and advising on all aspects of infection control.
- The ICN works with other trusts in matters relating to infection control as and when appropriate.
- The ICN formulates, contributes to and implements the trust's policies and guidelines relating to infection control with other members of the ICT and relevant staff.
- To evaluate, monitor and update infection control policies regularly throughout the trust, in accordance with recent research.
- To provide and evaluate education and training programmes on infection control for relevant health care workers working in the trust.
- To participate in the development and implementation of the annual programme for the hospital infection control committee.
- To provide advice and support to other ICNs working in the trust and, where appropriate, those of other trusts.
- To be actively involved in setting objectives for the provider unit ICNs and ensure that these are achieved.
- To establish and manage a team of ICLNs.
- To be involved in setting standards and monitoring and evaluating the infection control service across the trust.
- To promote safe working practices relating to infection control in accordance with the Health and Safety at Work Act (1974), COSHH Regulations (1994) and other relevant policies, including training of staff, investigation of, and reporting of hazardous or ineffective procedures.
- To participate in the surveillance of hospital acquired infection.

THE INFECTION CONTROL TEAM IN THE COMMUNITY

The NHS reforms in 1991 which separated the purchaser and provider have, as with most other specialties, had an impact on infection control nursing. The split originates from the NHS Community Care Act 1990. Purchasing, which is more correctly termed commissioning, is therefore still a relatively new concept within the NHS. One of the changes experienced by ICNs is that many used to cover both the hospital and community whereas now they only cover one provider trust. The shift from secondary to primary care provision has led to a reassessment of the role of the ICN in the community (this encompasses all areas outside the hospital).

The emergence of community infection control nurses (CICNs) who are employed by community provider trusts, public health departments and the Public Health Laboratory Service, and communicable disease control nurses (CDCNs) who work for the purchasers (the health authorities with the CCDC), has given recognition to the contribution of nurses to infection control in hospital and in the community. Their work is vital, challenging and exciting (DoH, 1995).

Community infection control nurses are specialist nurses who require an extensive general nursing experience, a background in community nursing and specialist knowledge of infection control. They may work for a number of different employees, as outlined above, and give advice to GPs, health visitors, residential and nursing homes, dentists, school nurses, local authorities, etc.

Community infection control nurse (CICN)

Qualifications and experience

The community infection control nurse should be a registered nurse, with a background in community nursing. For more senior posts they should have the diploma in infection control or equivalent, and should continue to remain up to date professionally once in post.

Accountability

The CICN is normally accountable to the consultant in communicable disease control, if working for a health authority or public health laboratory. If working for a community trust they may be accountable to the nurse advisor, medical director or a post specific to the trust.

Working relationships

The CICN works with:

- the consultant in communicable disease control (CCDC);
- other infection control teams;
- consultant microbiologists;
- staff of microbiology laboratories;
- the Public Health Laboratory Service;
- TB contact tracing nurses;
- the community nursing services;
- occupational health services;
- health promotion departments;
- primary health care staff;
- the Health and Safety Executive;
- local authority environmental health services;
- educational establishments;

- other agencies involved in the surveillance, prevention and control of infection in the district population.

Overall responsibilities

The CICN has to take the lead as specialist advisor on the surveillance, investigation and control of communicable disease within the health authority/trust area. He/she also has to develop research, standards and audit and risk management programmes to support the strategic development of infection control practice within health care establishments.

The role of the CICN

The role of the CICN includes the following activities:

- To develop, implement and monitor community infection control policies with the CCDC/other staff in the community trust.
- Serve as a member of the DICC and, as appropriate, attend meetings of committees and panels which deal with aspects of communicable disease control.
- Contribute to communicable disease needs assessment and participate in the work of the commissioning teams within the health authority.
- To develop and participate in education and training programmes on infection control for all disciplines and staff in the community.
- Assist in any annual reports.
- Take an active part in health promotion initiatives in relation to communicable disease prevention and control.
- To be a resource for the community of up to date, evidence-based information about infection control.
- Participate in the evaluation of current research and the appraisal of district policies and practices, making recommendations and implementing agreed change.
- Participate in appropriate research projects.
- If employed by the health authority, the CICN will work with the CCDC in the prevention, surveillance, and control of communicable diseases. She/he will assist local authority officers responsible for the receipt of infectious diseases notifications, collect and collate relevant clinical and epidemiological data, and participate in the surveillance of communicable diseases in the district.
- Assist in the management of individual cases and outbreaks of infection, e.g. meningitis, hepatitis B.
- To establish and maintain effective links with key personnel in the community.
- To establish and maintain links with other infection control teams and occupational health departments in trusts.

The consultant in communicable disease control (CCDC)

Qualifications and experience

The CCDC must be a registered medical practitioner formally trained in all aspects of communicable disease control. The CCDC has knowledge of the epidemiology of infectious disease, a knowledge of microbiology, management skills and an ability to communicate, liaise and collaborate. Most CsCDC are trained in public health medicine but some are microbiologists, infectious disease physicians and epidemiologists.

A higher qualification is desirable and this is usually membership of the Faculty of Public Health Medicine (MFPHM).

Accountability

The CCDC is accountable to the director of public health.

Working relationships

The CCDC works closely with hospital infection control doctors, agencies and professional groups concerned with infectious disease.

Overall responsibilities

The CCDC is usually appointed as the local authority's proper officer and performs duties relating to communicable diseases under the terms of the Local Government Act 1972, the Public Health (Control of Diseases) Act (1984) and Public Health (Infectious Disease) Regulations (1988).

The role of the CCDC

The role of the CCDC involves various activities as outlined below:

- The CCDC will have responsibility for establishing and maintaining monitoring systems that will enable effective surveillance of communicable disease within their HA. This involves working closely with infectious diseases clerks in environmental health departments. The CCDC also acts as medical adviser to local environmental health departments on matters relating to the control of communicable disease.
- The CCDC promotes understanding of effective mechanisms for the control and prevention of infection, and has a statutory responsibility to notify relevant personnel about specific certain diseases among doctors, nurses and the general population. He/she is responsible for the establishment of a rolling programme to maintain and improve the level of notification.

- Annual targets for the control of infectious diseases are another responsibility of the CCDC.
- The CCDC is responsible for the effective control of communicable disease. In the event of a major outbreak of infectious disease, the CCDC will be responsible for overall co-ordination of control of the outbreak, working closely with hospital infection control teams for control of infection in hospitals.
- The CCDC is responsible for ensuring that the appropriate persons notify diseases. When a potentially major outbreak of infection is suspected, the CCDC will inform the Communicable Disease Surveillance Centre, public health doctor on call and the appropriate doctor at the Department of Health if this is warranted.
- The CCDC is responsible for responding to the receipt of information that there is a suspected case of communicable disease within the health authority.
- The CCDC is responsible for maintaining up to date information on the incidence and prevalence of specific communicable diseases and to feed this information back to notifying doctors and to managers with responsibility for the control of communicable diseases.
- The CCDC contributes to the annual report for their population.
- The CCDC is a member of each provider trust infection control committee; ensuring consistent advice on matters relating to the control of communicable disease throughout the area.
- The CCDC ensures that there are effective major outbreak and control of infection procedures in place in his/her district.

The infection control link nurse (ICLN)

Many ICNs in hospital and the community have set up a system of infection control link nurses/midwives. In the hospital they are increasingly sited as facilitating liaison between clinical areas of the hospital and specialist teams for different aspects of medical care.

Qualifications and experience

ICLNs are first level nurses generally drawn from ward and departmental staff, with a minimum post-registration experience of two years, excluding any post-registration course.

Accountability

The ICLNs are accountable to their ward manager. However, they are responsible to the ICN in all matters related to infection control.

Working relationships

The ICLNs work with all members of the multidisciplinary team in their ward/department.

Overall responsibilities

Many ICNs throughout the UK have set up infection control link nurse/ midwife programmes in the belief that they will act as a resource in their particular clinical area and liaise with the ICT.

Role of the ICLN

The role of the ICLN involves various activities.

- To liaise between their clinical area and the ICT.
- To be directly responsible to the ICN with regard to the working of infection control policies and procedures in their clinical area.
- To liaise with the nurse in charge of the clinical area with regard to the implementation of infection control policies and procedures.
- In conjunction with the ICT, to act as a resource person for staff concerning infection control related problems in the clinical area (e.g. patient care practices, patient isolation and care of equipment).
- To assist in the education of staff in their clinical area in the principles of infection control as it relates to their specialty.
- To participate in the ICT/HICC activities as appropriate.
- To participate in the writing, reviewing and updating of infection control policies, procedures and standards in relation to their own specialty, as required by the ICN.
- To inform the ICN of any compromised and/or infected patient to ensure appropriate patient placement and precautions.
- To participate in teaching patients/staff appropriate aspects of care relating to infection control practices.
- To make surveillance rounds and keep accurate documentation. This will be done in conjunction with the ICT.
- To be knowledgeable regarding the purchase/introduction and use of equipment in their clinical area in relation to: infection control hazards; care and maintenance; decontamination and storage.
- To work in conjunction with the occupational health service on aspects related to infectious disease contact, needle/sharp injury exposure and follow-up, and COSHH regulations.
- To attend infection control link nurse meetings regularly.
- To take every opportunity to update and extend his or her knowledge of infection control.

This role, as described by the Department of Health and PHLS is very good. However, in practice, few if any full time staff on a normal busy ward doing internal rotation to night duty can commit themselves to attending the link nurse meetings regularly, let alone participate in surveillance and inform the ICT each time a patient with an infection is admitted. The ICTs cannot delegate these responsibilities to one nurse/midwife. If they are an effective ICT they should have communicated their infection control procedures to all staff and be undertaking surveillance themselves.

The environmental health officer (EHO)

The work of EHOs is extremely varied. The majority of EHOs are employed by local councils, and are employed to protect people living or working in their area. They can work in either generalised or specialised departments. Generalist EHOs are responsible for all aspects of environmental health in a particular area and specialists work alone or as part of a team responsible for a particular aspect of environmental health, such as food safety or noise pollution throughout the council's area. EHOs may also work for private industries, advising companies of their legal duties and helping them maintain good standards within the company. Other EHOs are employed by the Army, Navy and Air Force, universities and colleges. In the past few years some EHOs have become self-employed, working as consultants in both the private and public sectors.

Qualifications and experience

EHOs have a degree in Environmental Health.

Accountability

They are accountable through their local structure.

Working relationships

EHOs work with government departments, other departments, public authorities, outside organisations, companies and trade unions.

Overall responsibilities

The overall aim of the EHO is to reduce the risks and eliminate the dangers to human health associated with the living and working environment. This is achieved by inspecting premises, vehicles, plant, equipment, materials and persons; investigating complaints and infectious disease;

enforcing statutes applicable to the department; training and supervising staff; and undertaking health education.

The role of the EHO

The EHO is responsible for a variety of activities.

- To fulfil the council's statutory obligations in accordance with agreed policy and undertake the inspection and survey of premises, vehicles, stalls, plant, equipment, products, materials and plans.
- As an appointed inspector, under the Health and Safety at Work Act, the EHO is expected to serve prohibition and improvement notices and undertake enforcement, including the closure of premises, seizure of goods, articles and substances, when there are risks associated with human health and safety. EHOs are entitled to institute proceedings through the courts in their own name.
- To take executive decisions in the field in potentially dangerous or sensitive situations.
- To investigate, obtain, collect, collate, prepare, present and be personally responsible for case evidence for submission to the borough solicitor.
- To undertake the seizure and sampling of products and materials, some of a dangerous and toxic nature, in accordance with statutory procedures for analysis and testing with referral to expert agencies where necessary.
- In conjunction with the group officer, Principal Environmental Health Officer or Principal Environmental Services Officer to set personal work programmes within agreed priorities in order to undertake the investigation of complaints, contraventions of legislation or licensing requirements, infection, accidents and dangerous occurrences and other circumstances of environmental health significance.
- To initiate and undertake research or surveys related to the work of the department.
- To attend court at all levels, tribunals, public inquiry committees and give evidence in connection with the above duties.
- To provide specialist advice within the authority as required.
- To authorise and undertake the enforcement of other legislative or licensing requirements in accordance with delegated powers and responsibilities of the department.
- To be responsible for undertaking investigation in respect of infectious diseases and for liaising with appropriate medical personnel.
- To represent the division at council panels or working parties, public meetings, or public inquiries, as required.
- To be responsible for the maintenance and updating of records to provide statistical and procedural records.

- Be aware of day to day developments of new technology in analytical and monitoring equipment and the use of such equipment.
- To scrutinise, process and comment on statutory applications, planning applications and schemes when asked to give guidance.
- To undertake environmental health education work, both within and outside the department.
- To keep up to date with all relevant legislation, technical information, current policies and techniques appropriate to specific levels of responsibility.
- To train staff as appropriate, and be responsible for the supervision of students and other trainees as required.

THE FUTURE

With the health reforms and the growing emphasis on primary care, differentiation is emerging between the roles of nurses supporting CCDCs and those in trusts. However, it is vitally important to remember that effective infection control provision across diverse settings would benefit from local co-ordination of policies. Furthermore the role of the CCDC is expanding to include non-infectious environmental and chemical hazards. This will require closer working links with local occupational health units, agriculture and industry.

REFERENCES

Abel-Smith, B. (1964) *The Hospitals 1800–1948*, Heineman, London.

DoH/PHLS (1995) Hospital Infection Working Group of the Department of Health and PHLS. Hospital Infection Control Guidance on the Control of Infection In Hospitals. HSG (95) 10. *Tech. Rep.*

Gardner, A.M.N. and Oxon, B.M. (1962) The infection control sister: a new member of the control of infection team in general hospitals. *Lancet*, **2** (453), 710–11.

Health and Safety at Work Act (1974) HMSO, London.

DoH (1995) *Making it Happen Public Health – The Contribution, Role and Development of Nurses, Midwives and Health Visitors.* Report of the Standard Nursing and Midwifery Advisory Committee. BAPS, DoH, London.

Medical Research Council (1944) *The Control of Cross Infection in Hospitals*, War Memorandum No. 11, HMSO, London.

Ministry of Health: Central Health Services Council (1959) *Staphylococcal Infections in Hospitals*, Report of the Sub-Committee, HMSO, London.

Prieto, J. (1994) The specialist role of the ICN. *Nursing Times*, **90** (38), 63–5.

Public Health (Control of Diseases) Act (1984) HMSO, London.

Public Health (Infectious Diseases) Regulations (1988) HMSO, London.
The Control of Substances Hazardous to Health Regulations (COSHH) (1994)
SI 1994: 3246.

FURTHER READING

Lewis, J. (1995) The changing world of the community infection control nurse.
Healthy Alliance, 12–13.
RCN (1994) *Purchasing for health: a Royal College of Nursing guide*, RCN,
London.

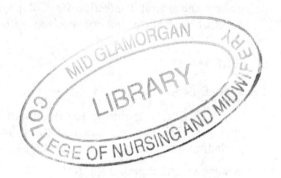

6 | The infection control committee (ICC)

The hospital ICT carries the prime responsibility for infection control and prevention. However it cannot work in isolation and requires the support of senior management, and other hospital staff. Every hospital should have a hospital infection control committee (HICC) (DoH/PHLS, 1995). The HICC will be the main forum for regular meetings to discuss and review the hospital infection control programme. The ICT will draw up most of the policies but requires the endorsement of the HICC.

THE HICC

Objectives

The HICC is responsible for developing standards, policies, procedures and guidelines on matters related to infection control in the hospital, including outbreak and major outbreak plans. In addition it:

- advises and supports the ICT;
- advises the chief executive of any serious infection control problems;
- acts as a source of expert advice on infection control to trust personnel;
- considers outbreak reports, and helps to implement recommendations;
- discusses and endorses the annual programme of infection prevention and control;
- promotes the education of all members of staff on infection control;
- has active involvement in auditing the infection control programme.

Membership of the HICC

Membership of the HICC includes:

- the ICT;
- the chief executive or a manager with authority to represent him or her;

- the CCDC for the health authority;
- occupational health representation;
- the infectious diseases physician, if not ICD;
- a consultant virologist;
- senior medical staff representing physicians and surgeons;
- the director of nursing or representative;
- representatives from any other hospitals covered by the HICC;
- clerical support.

The HICC should meet at least twice a year, ideally four times a year. The chairperson may invite other professionals to the meetings as appropriate, e.g. the local authority EHO, manager of the estates department, a pharmacist, or central sterile supplies manager. The HICC will normally be chaired by the ICD, and it is important that the HICC receives clerical support.

Meetings

Agendas

All members of the HICC should feel that they can contribute to the agenda. A typical meeting will cover the following:

- report(s) by the ICT on any outbreaks of infection that have occurred since the last meeting, and the HICC will endorse any appropriate recommendations made by the ICT;
- the need to write any new infection control policies;
- routine revision of existing infection control policies;
- budget requirements of the ICT;
- advice to other health care professionals on such aspects as building works, moving wards, closing off water supplies and tendering for contracts;
- supporting the ICT in any difficulties they may have encountered;
- reports from the district infection control committee;
- reports on the surveillance of hospital acquired infection.

Minutes

Minutes should be circulated to members of the HICC, and the hospital's chief executive, medical director and heads of directorates.

Policy documents

After any infection control policies have been approved by the HICC they should go to the chief executive for final ratification, particularly where there are financial implications. They should then become hospital policy and be implemented in accordance with the recognised process within the trust.

Emergency meetings

The chairperson or deputy may call an emergency meeting of the HICC when an outbreak of infection is suspected. If there is any community involvement then the CCDC will be invited to attend.

Community trusts

Many community trusts are appointing ICNs and are also organising their own ICCs. They support the infection control practitioners, ratify infection control policies, give advice on outbreak reports and act in a similar way to the HICC.

The DICC

The previous guidance on hospital infection control, issued in 1988, recommended that each district should have its own DICC (DHSS/PHLS, 1988). The new guidance, issued in 1995, accepts that each hospital should now have an HICC and that more and more provider units are setting up their own ICCs. As a consequence, CCDCs and ICTs could potentially be spending a lot of their time attending ICCs. However, they still feel that there is the need for a forum where ICTs from many different areas can come together and discuss infection control issues.

Objectives

The objectives of the DICC are:

- to review and provide advice on district wide infection control strategies and polices affecting several provider units;
- to enable collaboration between different provider units, the purchasers, local authorities and other agencies;
- to liaise with neighbouring DICCs;
- to assist the CCDC to provide advice to purchasers, providers, GPs, nursing and residential homes, etc.

Membership of the DICC

Membership of the DICC includes:

- ICDs and Senior ICNs from hospitals covered;
- community infection control practitioners;

- CCDC;
- director of public health;
- local authority representatives;
- water company representatives;
- immunisation co-ordinators;
- local education authority.

THE LOCAL HEALTH AUTHORITY

The health authority (HA) has a dual role in relation to infection control. As a purchaser of care for its population it wants to ensure the quality of the services. It is however directly responsible, with the local authorities, for protecting the public health by controlling communicable diseases, and managing environmental hazards. The responsibilities of the HA are met in the following ways:

- through contracts specifying infection control with the provider units;
- through the CCDC and their links with the ICTs;
- through the CCDC as their role as expert advisor to the HA;
- through the DICC.

Commissioning with provider units

The primary source of communicable disease control advice to the HA is the CCDC, or CICN. HSG(93)56, (DoH/DoE, 1993) states that communicable disease control should be taken into consideration in every contract between purchasing authorities and provider units.

The following are the four main objectives which the HA's contracts with the providers should encompass:

- effective arrangements for the protection of clients, health care workers and the general public from communicable disease and infection;
- to provide a basis for quality auditing of standards of infection control;
- to facilitate the providers to undertake their own surveillance, prevention and control of infection;
- to enable and safeguard the sharing of information between the CCDC, ICTs, laboratories and any other relevant people or organisations.

The HA would want the provider units to be setting their own standards and auditing their own achievement as described (Chapter 4). The following are the areas in which the HA would want to know that appropriate policies, personnel, programmes and audit systems are in place:

- compliance with statutory requirements, including the notification of certain infectious diseases, food hygiene, health and safety, waste management;

- following DoH guidance on such issues as hospital infection control, hepatitis B and immunisation;
- hospital outbreak and major outbreak plans;
- participation in the DICC and implementation of any related policies;
- the provision of adequately resourced HICTs and HICCs;
- an annual, reviewed infection control programme which goes through the HICC;
- an effective risk management system;
- an effective audit programme;
- sharing of information between provider units, the CCDC, laboratories and the DICC for the purposes of communicable disease control;
- supporting the CCDC during outbreaks of infection by providing laboratory services and staff.

GP FUNDHOLDERS

GP fundholders (GPFHs) are purchasers of some of the care for their patients. They are interested in the quality of the care their patients receive from provider units. HSG(93)56 (1993) advised GPFHs to collaborate with the HA in drawing up a shared and unified purchasing strategy with the HA which will bring about improvements in public health. Within the HA the best person for GPFHs to obtain advice from on local arrangements and provision of infection control is the CCDC.

REFERENCES

DoH/PHLS (1995) Hospital Infection Working Group of the Department of Health and Public Health Laboratory Service. *Hospital Infection Control Guidance on the Control of Infection in Hospitals.* HSG(95)10, BAPS, *Tech. Rep.*
Department of Health and Department of the Environment (1993) *Public Health: Responsibilities and the Roles of Others,* HSG(93)56, BAPS, *Tech. Rep.*
DHSS/PHLS (1988) *Hospital Infection Control: General Management Arrangements.* HC (88) 33, HMSO, London.

The statutory basis of infection control

7

In 1846, the Liverpool Sanitary Act gave authority for the appointment of the first Medical Officer of Health (MOH). This was Dr William Henry Duncan.

Subsequently, following the 1872 Act, and the formation of new local sanitary authorities, responsibility for the control of communicable disease was placed with these authorities and, by statute on the MOH. This situation continued until 26 years after the founding of the NHS when it and local government were reorganised in 1974.

Although the National Health Service Act had placed a generic responsibility on the Secretary of State to make provision for the prevention and treatment of illness, including the prevention and treatment of notifiable and other communicable diseases, statutory responsibility for communicable disease control remained with the local authority. Under the provisions of the Public Health Acts, it was discharged wholly by the MOH, who was a full time employee of the local authority.

These arrangements were changed considerably by the Local Government Act of 1972, and the National Health Service Reorganisation Act of 1973. When the provisions of these Acts came into force in 1974, the local authority post of MOH was abolished. However, the environmental health functions remained with local authorities, some as the responsibility of the authority itself, and some as the responsibility of officers of the authority, designated as 'proper officer' for this purpose.

Guidance on this division of responsibilities was issued jointly by the Department of Health and Social Services (DHSS) and the Department of the Environment (DoE) in circular HSC(73)74 (DHSS, 1973) immediately prior to the reorganisation of local government and the health service. It addressed the necessity of close collaboration between local and health authorities on the control of communicable disease. This circular, in paras 17 and 18, made it clear that the local authority should appoint as its medical adviser, the community physician of the health authority, who was a full time medical officer working in the NHS.

To enable such community physicians to act lawfully on behalf of the local authority these community physicians, who were to become known colloquially as the 'medical officer of environmental health (MOEHs)', were appointed as the proper officer for the Public Health Act, under section 162 of the Local Government Act.

As part of the basis of defining responsibilities under legislation, there is invariably a framework established to ensure that compliance with the legislation can be ensured. From the perspective of public health practitioners, enforcement is a final step which in many cases can be avoided. However there will always be those who, for their own interests, deliberately flout their reponsibilities, and mandatory enforcement becomes necessary.

THE ROLE OF ENFORCEMENT AGENCIES IN CONTROL OF INFECTION

Infection control in the health care environment is usually, although not always, the responsibility of the Health and Safety Executive. However infection control in its broadest sense, covers a far wider range of activities than those occurring in designated health care establishments, such as hospitals or general practice surgeries.

A number of important Acts have relevance to communicable disease control at an environmental level, and relate largely to ensuring the safety of the infrastructure of the environment. For example, the provision of drains and sewers, and ensuring there are sufficient sanitary conveniences, is one such area; regulations relating to these are contained in the Public Health Acts of 1936 and 1961.

The Environmental Protection Act, 1990, contains provisions governing the disposal of waste, including clinical waste, and places a duty of care on producers. Waste regulation authorities (WRAs), waste disposal authorities, and waste collection authorities are established under the Act and associated regulations. In general, waste regulation authorities are the county councils, although in London, Manchester and Liverpool there are separate authorities, e.g. in London, the London waste regulation authority.

The Food Safety Act, 1990, provides a legislative framework to ensure the safety of food from infectious agents, by ensuring compliance with general food hygiene regulations.

Enforcement agencies

The term communicable disease control covers the prevention, surveillance, investigation and control of all communicable diseases. While overall responsibility for communicable disease control is divided between health and local authorities, the statutory powers under the 1984 Act rest with the local authority. Other legislation moreover provides powers and responsibilities to a range of related activities relevant to infection control. For example, the inspection of premises and the hygienic control of food and water and the control of other environmental vehicles of infection such as the safe disposal of sharps and other clinical waste, are accepted as essential components of the management of communicable disease. It is important to be clear that agencies outside the NHS and local authority EHOs also fulfil a role as enforcers of safety and other public health legislation.

ACTS AND REGULATIONS

Health and Safety at Work Act 1974 (HSAWA)

Health and safety at work is an area that is sometimes seen as an expensive extra, rather than an essential part of corporate strategy that will improve efficiency and business performance. Until 1991, under Crown Immunity, the NHS was exempt, but the removal of Crown Immunity has brought about an improved focus of NHS management to health and safety issues.

In June 1996, under cover of EL(96)44, the NHS management executive sent out a circular letter on health and safety in the NHS (DoH, 1996), emphasising the need for effective management, and restating the commitment of the NHSME to ensure that health and safety would be seen as an important aspect in the NHS. The letter contains useful information, reporting that the following prosecutions occurred in the health sector between 1993 and 1995 (Table 7.1).

Health risk management today is about identifying and controlling risks before they cause problems and lead to injury. Compliance with the HSAWA at the most basic level requires that any employer employing more than five employees must operate an up to date written health and safety policy, carry out a risk assessment, record the main findings and arrangements for health and safety, and report certain diseases. Section 18(7)(a) of the Act defines the enforcing authority as 'the Executive (HSE) or any other authority which is by relevant statutory provision or by regulation . . . made responsible for the enforcement of any of the provisions to any extent'. Thus, there is a division of responsibilities created which can sometimes be confusing, and which does not always appear to be applied logically. In addition, regulation 5 of the Act allows for the transfer of enforcement responsibility, either way, between HSE and LAs by mutual agreement.

Within the remit of infection control, the enforcement role is divided

Table 7.1 The number of prosecutions in the health care sector which have occurred between 1993 and 1995

Year	Act	Section	Totals
1993	RIDDOR	3(1)	1
	HSAWA	3(1)	2
		2(1)	2
	COSHH	6(1)	1
		7(1)	1
		12(1)	1
1994	RIDDOR	3	5
	HSAWA	3	6
	COSHH	12	1
1995	HSAWA	3(1)	7
	Manual Handling Regulations		1

between the HSE and local authority. Broadly speaking, the two agencies have a different approach to the problems. In general, the HSE places a greater emphasis on ensuring the safety of the environment, while LAs place a greater emphasis on their enforcement procedures.

In general, the HSE is responsible for enforcement in the health care environment, such as hospitals and GP surgeries. However, there are many activities that have an important infection control aspect for which they are not responsible, and control of the following areas falls to the local authorities.

- The use of a bath, sauna or solarium, hair transplanting, skin piercing, manicuring or other cosmetic service and therapeutic treatments, except where they are carried out under the supervision of a registered medical practitioner, a dentist registered under the Dentists Act 1984, a physiotherapist, an osteopath or a chiropractor.
- The activities of an undertaker, except where the main activity is embalming or the making of coffins.

Sometimes, uncertainty exists as to exactly which agency is responsible for enforcement responsibilities in the area between clearly non-medical work, such as hairdressing on the one hand, and the fully fledged hospital on the other. For example, a lack of clarity occurs with regard to nursing homes, that are registered by the health authority in which they are sited. A nursing home may carry out activities ranging from minimal care of the elderly, through to a maternity home or abortion clinic, or a fully operational health care unit which operates in a manner identical to an NHS hospital. While the HSE is technically responsible, in practice local authority officers will advise on much of this work.

It is not uncommon to find that many NHS employees are unaware that the Health and Safety at Work Act applies not only to employers and employees, but that section 3 of the Act places a responsibility on the employer to ensure the safety of others.

Control of Substances Hazardous to Health (COSHH) Regulations, 1988

The COSHH regulations, 1988 (SI, 1987) came into force on 1 October 1988, with an additional period until 1 October 1990 to allow for completion of the required assessments. The legislation rationalised or repealed dozens of highly specific but dated legislation. Indeed in a similar way to the HSAWA, this legislation applied general principles, in particular the principle of assessment, to outline what should be good working practices.

Employers should not undertake work that exposes employees to hazardous substances unless they make a 'suitable and sufficient assessment of risks'. These assessments must also be reviewed on a regular basis. It is not always intuitively understood that COSHH regulations apply to biological hazards in the workplace, as well as chemical and toxic hazards.

Laboratory workers handling cultures of pathogenic micro-organisms, and health care workers treating patients with infectious diseases are obviously at risk. Humans and their tissues can be a source of important occupational diseases for example, hepatitis B, tuberculosis, and HIV infection.

Risk assessment may be complex, because infection is not a straightforward process. It depends on the infecting dose, survival of the organism in the environment, the resistance and immune status of the host, and the possibility of secondary spread should a primary infection occur. Organisms have however been classified into four groupings.

- Group I: unlikely to cause disease.
- Group II: may cause disease, spread unlikely, treatment available.
- Group III: severe disease possible, spread possible.
- Group IV: severe disease probable, high risk of spread, treatment/ prophylaxis not normally available.

The Advisory Committee on Dangerous Pathogens (ACDP) specifies four containment levels corresponding to the above four hazard groupings (Table 7.2).

Table 7.2 Definitions of 4 hazard groups

Hazard group 1	An organism that is most unlikely to cause human disease.
Hazard group 2	An organism that might cause human disease and which might be a hazard to laboratory workers, but is unlikely to spread to the community. Laboratory exposure rarely produces infection and effective prophylaxis or effective treatment is usually available.
Hazard group 3	An organism that causes severe human disease and presents a serious hazard to laboratory workers. It may present a risk of spread to the community but there is usually effective prophylaxis or treatment available.
Hazard group 4	An organism that causes severe human disease and is a serious hazard to laboratory workers. It may present a high risk of spread to the community and there is usually no effective prophylaxis or treatment.

Reporting of Injuries, Diseases and Dangerous Occurrences, 1985 (as amended 1992)

The prevention of work related disease requires not only the effective control of the work environment but also good information about its incidence. These regulations, effective since 1985, and known as RIDDOR, provide the legislative background for the surveillance of work related disease. They require an employer to report to the Health and Safety Executive, work related incidents in the following categories.

- Notifiable accidents: acute illness requiring medical treatment when there is reason to believe that this resulted from exposure to a pathogen or infected material.
- Dangerous occurrences: accidental release of a biological agent likely to cause severe human illness (HSE, 1985).
- Certain diseases if an employee develops a reportable disease and works in a listed occupation.

These listed diseases must be reported on form F2509A forthwith following diagnosis by the medical practitioner.

While this provision refers mainly to occupationally acquired diseases, such as asthma, byssinosis, extrinsic alveolitis, pneumoconiosis and asbestos related cancers, there are several infectious diseases which are also included.

Leptospirosis

If the worker is an animal handler (e.g. medical research).

Hepatitis

If the work involves any exposure to human blood products, or body secretions and excretions.

Tuberculosis

If the work involves contact with persons or animals or with human or animal remains, or with any other material which might be a source of infection.

Other illnesses

Any illness caused by work involving a pathogen which presents a hazard to human health. The listed diseases must be reported on Form F2590A forthwith, following diagnosis by the medical practitioner. The responsible person in relation to these reports and notifications is normally the employer, or the person undertaking the training of someone undergoing training.

It is proposed that the current arrangements for reporting to the enforcing authority for the premises or work activity (i.e. HSE or LA) will be replaced by a national telephone reporting system which, when in place, will no longer require written confirmation. The system would bring all notifications to a central bureau and information would then be passed to the appropriate enforcing authority.

Notification of Cooling Towers and Evaporative Condensers Regulations, 1992

Notification of all cooling towers and evaporative condensers is required to be made to the LA in whose area the premises are situated, unless:

- no water is exposed to air;
- either the water or electricity supply are not connected.

These regulations serve two purposes. First, they allow the LA to monitor the environmental control of the installation, to ensure that effective maintenance practices are in place with regard to the prevention of Legionnaires' disease and, second, they enable a rapid check to be made of all such devices in the area should an outbreak of Legionnaires' disease occur. Notification has to be made in writing, and any changes to the notification particulars must be updated within one month of any material change.

Food Safety Act, 1990

The main provisions of the Food Safety Act (1990) came into force on 1 January 1991. Local authorities are the enforcing authorities for this legislation. All food business are required to be registered with the LA, and the Act provides for the detention and seizure of food suspected of not complying with food safety requirements.

Section 1 of the Act defines 'food' and other basic expressions used, such as 'food business', 'food premises' and 'food source'. Sections 7 and 8 describe the offence of rendering food injurious to health, and the offence of selling food that does not comply with food safety requirements. Improvement notices may be served when food hygiene of processing regulations have been breached, and where there is an immediate threat to safety, and there is provision for emergency prohibition.

Offences under the Act may result in serious penalties. For most offences a Crown Court may impose a prison sentence of up to two years or unlimited fines. Magistrates courts may impose fines of up to £2 000 and a prison sentence of up to six months. For the most serious offences a magistrates court may impose fines of up to £20 000.

Local Government (Miscellaneous Provisions) Act, 1982

Skin piercing

Under the Local Government (Miscellaneous Provisions) Act 1982, a LA may adopt provisions in respect of its own area. The skin piercing procedures which may be controlled by registration and application of local by-laws include:

- acupuncture;
- tattooing;
- ear piercing;
- electrolysis.

If such a business is carried on under the supervision of a registered medical practitioner, then there is no requirement to register. If not, then both the operator and the premises must be registered. A LA operating these procedures may make by-laws relating to the cleanliness of the premises and of persons working there, and with regard to the cleansing and sterilisation of instruments, materials and equipment.

Water safety

In England and Wales, legal and administrative arrangements are contained in the Water Act (1989), now consolidated in the Water

(Industry) Act 1991 which lays the responsibility for drinking water quality on the Secretary of State for the Environment.

Water supplied has to meet the standards laid down in the Water Quality Regulations and, to achieve this, water undertakers are obliged to take samples, test them and report the results to the local authority, the appropriate health authority and the Inspectorate, to make sure water meets these standards. Originally, these regulations applied only to water supplied for domestic purposes – that is for drinking, washing and cooking, but following amendments made to the Water Act by the Food Safety Act 1990, the Water Quality Regulations have been extended by the Water Supply (Water Quality) Amendment Regulations 1991 and now also apply to water used for food production.

Private water supplies also exist, and regulation to ensure that the water used is safe are contained in the Private Water Supplies Regulations, 1991, which came into force on 1 January 1992. Under these regulations, local authorities now have a statutory duty to sample and analyse private water supplies, to provide protection to people consuming water from these supplies or consuming food produced using such water supplies.

8	# Surveillance

The word 'surveillance' means different things to different people. If asked to define surveillance many would think of it as being watched, for example by the police, or closed circuit television, without any obvious benefits to the person under surveillance. Within the context of this book surveillance means the collection, collation, analysis and dissemination of information related to health. Surveillance is essential for the early identification of outbreaks or potential outbreaks in both the hospital and community. Surveillance is conducted at international, national and local level through a wide range of systems, and by many different organisations.

HISTORY OF SURVEILLANCE

England was one of the first countries in the world to conduct surveillance, though not necessarily for the good of the population at large. The Bills of Mortality, which began in the sixteenth century recorded the reasons why people died in the City of London. This enabled the court to leave London when plague was rife. In 1889 the statutory notification system came into being, but the system is not generally well understood by the medical profession. Under section 10 of the Public Health (Control of Disease) Act a legal duty is placed on every registered medical practitioner once he/she:

'becomes aware or *suspects* that a patient whom he is attending within the district of a local authority is suffering from a notifiable disease or from food poisoning, he shall unless he believes, and has reasonable grounds for believing, that some other registered medical practitioner has complied with this subsection with respect to this patient, forthwith send to the proper officer of the local authority for that district a certificate stating' a limited number of personal data items.

This report should be made on a prescribed form, that has to comply with the general layout specified in the Act, and these are supplied by the local authority free of charge to all registered medical practitioners in their district (Figure 8.1).

Although the notification form is sent to the local authority, it is the health authority that is responsible for paying to the registered medical practitioner a fee (currently £2.30) for each certificate. The notification form is a confidential document, and there is therefore a duty for it to be sent in such a manner that its contents cannot be read during transmission, and the information contained therein shall not be divulged to any person except: so far as is necessary for compliance with the requirements of any enactment (including the Regulations), or for the purposes of such action as any proper officer considers reasonably necessary for preventing the spread of disease.

It is one of the few situations in which a medical practitioner is obliged to breach medical confidentiality. The details to be notified must include:

- the name, age and sex of the patient;
- the address of the patient;
- the disease or suspected disease;
- the date of onset of illness;
- and, if the patient is in hospital, the address from which the person came, and an opinion as to whether the disease was contracted in the hospital.

All medical staff have a statutory duty to notify the relevant proper officer of the local authority of certain infectious diseases and food poisoning when diagnosed, or suspected, in patients they are attending Table 8 1 All the powers and procedures for the notification and control of notifiable diseases are enforced by the local authority and are formally delegated by the council of the local authority to an officer known as the proper officer. The proper officer is 'that officer nominated for that purpose'. In England and Wales the proper officer is usually the consultant in communicable disease control (CCDC). In Scotland and Northern Ireland this role is undertaken by the chief administrative medical officer (CAMO) or director of public health. When so appointed, the CCDC or CAMO is responsible to the local authority (and not the health authority) when exercising any of these delegated powers.

When this system was first introduced at the end of the nineteenth century telephones and faxes were obviously not available, and so the formal notifications were sent by post on a standard form. Books of the forms are provided by the local authority or health authority to all hospitals and general practitioners in their area (Figure 8.1). However, today, proper officers generally expect suspected urgent cases to be reported immediately, without waiting for laboratory confirmation of the cause, by telephone, fax, or even modem. Written notification on the standard certificate should follow as soon as possible.

NOTIFICATION OF INFECTIOUS DISEASE OR FOOD POISONING

No:

SURNAME	DATE OF BIRTH	DISEASE (see note on cover)	DATE OF ONSET	OCCUPATION
FORENAME	SEX: MALE/FEMALE			

Full address of where patient is now:

If the patient is at present in hospital, the address in full from which the patient was admitted is:
....
....
....

Tel. no. (home):

Ethnic origin (see note on cover):

In my opinion, the disease was/was not contracted abroad (delete whichever does not apply)

MALARIA — Parasitic type: — Where contracted:

MENINGITIS — Viral/bacterial/other:
Causal organism, if known:

ACUTE POLIOMYELITIS — please circle the appropriate type — Paralytic — Non-paralytic

TUBERCULOSIS — Organ or part affected: — Sputum smear positive – YES/NO:
BCG given in past – YES/NO: — If 'YES', when?   /   /

I believe this case to be linked with other cases of similar disease – YES/NO: — Specimen sent for examination – YES/NO
If 'YES', please give details: .... — Type of specimen:

I hereby certify and declare that in my opinion the person named above is suffering — Result (if any) of examination............................
from the disease stated
Signature of doctor:.................. Date: /   /

Name of doctor (please PRINT):...............

Name and address of GP (if different):
....
....
....

Postal address of practice/hospital/department:
....
....
....

Figure 8.1 Example of a form for notification of an infectious disease

Table 8.1 Diseases notifiable to the proper officer

England and Wales

Acute encephalitis	Opthalmia neonatorum
Acute poliomyelitis	Paratyphoid fever
Anthrax	Plague
Cholera	Rabies
Diphtheria	Relapsing fever
Food poisoning (or	Rubella
suspected food poisoning)	Scarlet fever
Lassa fever	Smallpox
Leptospirosis	Tetanus
Leprosy	Tuberculosis (all forms)
Malaria	Typhoid fever
Measles	Typhus
Meningitis	Viral haemorrhagic fever (e.g. Ebola)
Meninococcal septicaemia	Viral hepatitis
(without meningitis)	Whooping cough
Mumps	Yellow fever

Scotland

Anthrax	Scarlet fever
Chickenpox	Smallpox
Cholera	Tetanus
Diphtheria	Tuberculosis – respiratory non-respiratory
Dysentery	Plague
Erysipelas	Poliomyelitis – paralytic and non-paralytic
Food poisoning	Puerperal fever
Legioncllosis	Rabies
Leptospirosis	Relapsing fever
Leprosy	Rubella
Malaria	Typhoid fever
Measles	Typhus
Meningococcal infection	Viral haemorrhagic fevers (e.g. Ebola)
Mumps	Viral hepatitis
Paratyphoid fever A and B	Whooping cough

Northern Ireland

Acute encephalitis	Plague
Acute meningitis	Poliomyelitis – paralytic and non-paralytic
Anthrax	Rabies
Chickenpox	Relapsing fever
Cholera	Rubella
Diphtheria	Scarlet fever
Dysentery	Smallpox
Food poisoning (all sources)	Tetanus
Gastro-enteritis (under two years of age only)	Tuberculosis – pulmonary and
Hepatitis A, B and unspecified viral	non-pulmonary
Legionnaires' disease	Typhoid fever
Leptospirosis	Typhus
Malaria	Viral haemorrhagic fevers
Measles	Whooping cough
Mumps	Yellow fever
Paratyphoid fever	

Proper officers are required, under the Public Health (Infectious Diseases) Regulations (1988), to inform the health departments of England and Wales immediately about any of the following diseases:

- cholera;
- plague;
- smallpox;
- yellow fever.

In addition, in England and Wales, CsCDC are requested to inform the director of the Communicable Disease Surveillance Centre by telephone of any large, unusual, institutional or serious outbreak of foodborne illness. In Scotland, consultants in public health medicine (CPHMs) are required to inform the Scottish Home and Health Department of any serious outbreaks, and are also requested to inform the Scottish Centre for Infections and Environmental Health. In Northern Ireland the DHSS should be informed of any outbreaks through the chairman of the Communicable Diseases Liaison Group.

Anonymous returns of data derived from notifications are sent weekly by the local authority to the Office of National Statistics (ONS, formerly OPCS).

SURVEILLANCE

Laboratory reporting

Laboratories analysing samples from patients or other environmental samples also have an important role to play in identifying outbreaks. This is however an informal system. The PHLS has a responsibility to assist in the identification or management of outbreaks of infection. Other microbiologists, either in the NHS or private, may report results of public health importance informally to the proper officer/CCDC. In some areas this system has been updated so that the computers in the proper officer's office and the reporting laboratories are linked electronically enabling rapid data transfer.

General public

The general public also have a role to play in reporting infectious diseases and foodborne illness. They may complain to the environmental health department of the local authority regarding a restaurant or snack bar they have used which they felt was unsatisfactory, or if they have been ill through eating potentially contaminated food. This is an important source of information that is often unrecognised. Many healthy adults do not visit their GP if they are unwell with an infectious disease or potential foodborne illness, and this reporting to the local authority is one way of addressing this lack of data.

Data collection

Within the UK both the health authorities, or health boards, and local authorities collect surveillance data. Data is also collected nationally (Figure 8.1; Table 8.1). Interpretation is usually undertaken by the health authorities. It is important that all organisations that collect data are aware of the data being collected elsewhere to avoid duplication of work and to ensure that all data provided is meaningful.

In hospitals

Surveillance is an essential component for the prevention and control of infection in hospitals and consists of the routine collection, tabulation, analysis and dissemination of the resulting information to those who need to know so that appropriate action can be taken (DoH, 1995). Much of the information that should be available on the hospital information system, and inpatient hospital notes is very poorly recorded and often incomplete (Emmerson et al., 1996). The two main objectives of hospital surveillance are:

- the prevention and early detection of hospital outbreaks;
- the assessment and comparison of infection levels over a period of time so that the need for and effect of infection control measures can be seen.

For surveillance to be effective, it is essential that it is seen as part of the routine work of the clinical teams working in the hospital. The HICC must be seen as the area where expert advice on the surveillance of hospital acquired infection is available. If surveillance is to be adopted as an integral part of health care, the clinical teams in the hospital have to have ownership of surveillance programmes relating to their area. This is because they understand their area better than any one else and are aware of any potential areas of improvement. If surveillance results are fed back to HCWs who have had little or no input into the surveillance programme, they may find fault with the programme or simply not act on the results. The ICT must be seen as the infection control experts to give advice on, not run surveillance programmes. In many areas surveillance by the infection control teams is still very much in its infancy, and it may be some considerable time before clinical teams begin to have their own surveillance programmes. The national prevalence study conducted in 1993/4 was seen by many ICNs as very time consuming (Emmerson et al., 1996), and many ICTs are undertaking selective surveillance as this appears to be the most appropriate use of current resources. Many health authorities expect their provider units to undertake surveillance on the basis that it will lead to improvements in practice aimed at preventing avoidable infections. However purchasers should be cautious in their expectations of and use of surveillance programmes.

Undertaking surveillance

Before an infection control team begins to consider undertaking surveillance they must answer the following questions.

- What is the purpose of the surveillance? Will the results affect patient care?
- Who will organise the surveillance process?
- Are the appropriate clinicians interested in surveillance?
- Is the data to be collected already collected by another department/ organisation?
- If the data is not already available who will collect the data?
- Who will analyse the data?
- Who will interpret the data?
- Who will fund the surveillance?
- Who will write the final report, and where will it go?
- How will the effect of the surveillance be measured?
- Are they going to conduct a prevalence or incidence study?

Once they are happy with answers to the above they need to write out a detailed protocol, and consider the need for ethical approval. All surveillance methods have the following key components:

- data collection using case definitions;
- collation of data;
- analysis and interpretation of data;
- dissemination of information for action to those who need to know.

Data collection and case definitions

Data collected will depend in many incidences on the data available. Data items commonly used include:

- patient/person identifier;
- age;
- sex;
- area;
- date of admission/discharge;
- onset of symptoms;
- dates and types of invasive procedures;
- antibiotics used;
- organisms isolated.

Surveillance is used most frequently with the most common types of noscomial infections, e.g. urinary tract infections, surgical wound infections, respiratory tract and bloodstream infections. Depending on the type of surveillance being undertaken, further details will be added to these topics. For example, surgical wound infection rates can be categorised into operative procedure, surgeon and length of time on the operating table. It is also generally accepted that there are other risk factors involved in surgery, e.g. if someone is over 65 years, or has three or more other underlying medical problems, they are more likely to acquire an infection. In the hospital setting much of the above information is already available, computerised on the hospital information systems, e.g. patient administration system, operating theatre system and pathology department system. Computer programmes are available which can link the many different hospital information systems in place so that much of the data need only be collected and entered once.

Much of the data that are seen to be important for surveillance are already available. A representative from the local information technology department is therefore a very valuable addition to any surveillance working group, as they will know how to link systems and how to analyse data. They will also be more familiar with the many different computer programmes available for the collation and analysis of data. Where a lot of data are available, information on the overall infection rate in a whole hospital is difficult to interpret, and therefore of doubtful value. It is more effective to develop year on year comparisons of the data in the hospital, making allowances for changes in practice.

Also, if the results of surveillance are to be compared it is imperative that agreed case definitions are used.

When collecting data, particularly in the hospital it is important to realise that many people develop an infection in the community. This is because escalating medical costs in the 1990s and the introduction of day-care surgery have resulted in shorter hospital stays and higher volumes of outpatient surgical procedures. This makes it extremely difficult to calculate HAI surgical wound infection rates. A number of studies have highlighted the problem. Byrne *et al.* (1994), found that, with careful post-discharge surveillance and attention to definitions of infection, some 60% of post-operative wound infections occurred after discharge.

Analysis and interpretation of data

Routine surveillance data should be carefully examined, ideally daily, to detect unexpected clustering of cases. Undertaking a large surveillance project and only looking at the results at the end of three or four months may result in lost potential for preventing the spread of infection. If infection rates are being examined then numerator and denominator data must be used. Different data types may be used for the numerator, e.g. the number of infected patients or the number of patients, and for the denominator, from patient days, consultant episodes, deaths or length of inpatient stay. These will give different rates of infection, and it is important that the infection control practitioners are aware that their surveillance data will be looked at by many different people and could be misused. Therefore, it is vital that informed professional advice is used to interpret the results. This is due to the inevitable differences in case-mix in different hospitals. Two types of studies may be undertaken, either a 'prevalence' or 'incidence' study. A prevalence study will show the total number of cases of infections in existence in a given population at a certain time: it is a 'snapshot' study. An incidence study will show the number of new infections which occur over a period of time, for example the number of cases of measles in a year.

Dissemination of information

The feedback of information to the appropriate medical and nursing staff is an essential component of any surveillance programme. It has been shown that the dissemination of information to clinical teams leads to a reduction in infection rates (Haley et al., 1985). Surveillance can also be used for audit, as the information will help clinical staff with this. The results of surveillance should be reported regularly to the HICC and risk management committee. Surveillance must be seen to be open and explicit.

The true 'incidence' of hospital acquired infection (HAI) in the UK and Republic of Ireland is not known. A national 'prevalence' study conducted in 1993/94 showed the prevalence of HAI to be 9.0% (Emmerson et al., 1996). In the United States many hospitals participate in the national nosocomial infections surveillance system, which began in 1970, when the centers for disease control and prevention (CDC) invited selected hospitals to report routinely their nosocomial infection surveillance data for aggregation into a national data base. It is the only source of national data on the epidemiology of nosocomial infections in the USA. A similar programme is beginning in England and Wales, which will provide national data on nosocomial infections.

REFERENCES

Byrne, D.J., Lynch, W., Napier, A., et al. (1994) Wound infection rates: the importance of definition and post-discharge wound surveillance. *Journal of Hospital Infection*, **26**, 37–43.
Department of Health (1995) *Hospital Infection Control; guidance on the control of*

infection in hospitals, prepared by the hospital infection working group of the Department of Health and Public Health Laboratory Service, BAPS, Lancashire.

Emmerson, A.M., Enstone, J.E., Griffin, M., Kelsey, M.C. and Smyth, E.T.M. (1996) The second national prevalence survey of infection in hospitals – overview of the results. *Journal of Hospital Infection*, **32**, 175–90.

Hayley, R.W., Culver, D.H., White, J.W., *et al.* (1985) The efficacy of infection surveillance and control programs in preventing nosocomial infection in US hospitals. *American Journal of Epidemiology*, **121**, 182.

<table>
<tr><td>9</td><td># Universal infection control precautions (UICPs)</td></tr>
</table>

| 9 | **Universal infection control precautions (UICPs)** |

Universal infection control precautions (UICPs) or universal precautions are familiar terms to most health care workers in the 1990s. There is however, considerable confusion surrounding the definition of UICPs, and they are usually seen as a way of preventing the spread of infection among the population in a hospital or the community. UICPs are, in fact, a template principle on which all appropriate infection control precautions should be based.

HISTORY AND DEVELOPMENT

In 1983, as a result of the fear surrounding the disease AIDS (acquired immunodeficiency syndrome) the centers for disease control (CDC) in the US published the document *Blood and Body Fluid Precautions in Hospitals* (Garner and Simmons, 1983). These initial guidelines recommended that health care workers should practise blood and body fluid precautions *only* when they knew or suspected a patient of being infected with blood borne pathogens. This inevitably created a certain level of confusion and discrimination in the health care setting as an extra level of precautions was added to the other forms of barrier nursing already being practised, e.g. enteric and respiratory precautions. Staff did not necessarily understand why they were taking these extra precautions and a lot of unnecessary fear and worry was created.

In 1987, the CDC published a further document which recommended consistent use of blood and body fluid precautions for all patients, irrespective of their blood borne infection status. In the context of this document, UICPs referred to blood and certain other body fluids and tissues which were considered potentially infectious for the human immunodeficiency virus (HIV) and hepatitis B (HBV).

While acknowledging the 1987 CDC guidelines, many infection control practitioners have taken the concept further with the aim of educating all HCWs so that they follow consistent infection control precautions when exposed to all body fluids. If these precautions are followed they will protect both the HCWs and their clients/patients from most infections, not just blood borne infections, but others transmitted by faeces and urine, such as hepatitis A, salmonella and cytomegalovirus (CMV). This consistent use of universal infection control precautions means that there is no need to change the infection control precautions being practised once an infection is identified. For example, if precautions such as glove wearing are always taken whenever a HCW may come into contact with excreta, there will be no need for any extra precautions once a person is found to have an infection spread by faeces such as typhoid fever.

In health care, the safest and simplest way of defining UICPs is to acknowledge that blood and body fluids may contain blood borne viruses (e.g. hepatitis B, C and HIV) or other bacterial or viral pathogens (e.g. salmonella and CMV) which can present a risk to other patients and staff. As it is not always possible to know who is infected with these pathogens, and so there are certain precautions which must be taken with blood and most body fluids at all times.

There is no doubt that HCWs and patients are at risk, particularly from blood borne viruses. In areas where the prevalence of hepatitis B (HBV) in the general population is low (Australia, North America and Western Europe) fewer than 1% of patients are found to carry HBV. In these areas however the prevalence of HBV in HCWs is reported to be 5 to 10 times greater than in the general population, presumably as a result of occupational exposure.

The former categorisation of blood and/or body fluids when defining UICP into fluids which may contain blood borne viruses and those which may contain other pathogenic micro-organisms was complex and difficult to remember, and therefore often not followed.

A strong recommendation today is that for UICP to be followed they need to be simple, easy to understand and to be applied in the care of all patients/clients at all times. The infection control precautions outlined below when used routinely minimise the spread of potential pathogens from staff to clients, client to client and client to staff.

THE LEGAL FRAMEWORK OF UICP IN THE UK

COSHH

In the UK, under the Health and Safety at Work Act (1974) and the Control of Substances Hazardous to Health (COSHH) Regulations, 1988 and 1994, require all employers to evaluate risks to health for all their employees from exposure to hazardous substances at work. For this reason, a risk assessment programme is essential in the health environment for employers to identify what threatens health and safety and to evaluate the necessary measures to ensure they are safeguarded. Although most provider units recognise they must undertake a COSHH assessment when toxic chemicals are being used, e.g. glutaraldehyde or anaesthetic gases, it is not often acknowledged that COSHH specifically includes the risks from biohazards such as blood and body fluids which may contain pathogenic micro-organisms. The regulations require a risk assessment for the exposure and measures that are to be taken to limit exposure. Such risk assessments must be available to anyone performing that particular procedure.

UICPs are based on risk assessment and by basing infection control practice on UICP provider units, general practices and dental practices are helping to implement COSHH in the workplace. Indeed infection control is a requirement of the duty of care of all registered dentists (GDC, 1993).

UNDERSTANDING AND IMPLEMENTING UICP

The following principles are included in the implementation of universal infection control precautions:

- handwashing and drying;
- protective clothing;
- safe handling and disposal of sharps;
- spillages;
- environmental factors;
- isolation precautions.

Handwashing

Most people accept the need for handwashing, and social handwashing is one of the simplest methods of reducing the risk of cross-infection, by significantly reducing the carriage of potential pathogens on the hands in all settings including the home (Steere and Mallison, 1975; Sanderson and Weissler, 1992). The hands of staff are the most common vehicle by which micro-organisms are transmitted between patients and have frequently been implicated as the route of transmission of outbreaks of infection (Reybrouck, 1983; Casewell and Phillips, 1977). Unfortunately compliance with handwashing has been recognised as poor since the days of Semmelweis in the mid-nineteenth century, and still continues to be poor despite the invention of handwashing machines (Wurtz, Moye and

Jovanovic, 1994) and the recognition that it is central to the control of infection in the hospital and the community (Larson, 1988). Hospital staff members overestimate the frequency with which they wash their hands, as well as the duration of handwashing (Gould, 1995). HCWs wash their hands after touching patients with bare hands less than 50% of the time (Lund *et al.*, 1994, McLane *et al.*, 1983; Broughall *et al.*, 1984). However, other factors such as work load and very importantly the placing and accessibility of hand-wash basins, soap and hand towels may also play an important role in why HCWs do not always wash their hands as often as advocated in the literature.

Handwashing terminology

'Resident flora' is a term which describes micro-organisms persistently isolated from the skin of most people. These micro-organisms are considered to be permanent residents of the skin and indeed are necessary for people to remain healthy. They are not readily removed by handwashing.

'Transient flora' are microbes which people acquire on the surface of their skin from contact with other people, objects and their environment. These bacteria or viruses are not a normal part of the person's normal skin flora and are a potential cross-infection hazard. The composition of the transient flora a person carries on their hands varies as it is dependent on the amount of contact the person is having with other people and the environment and the prevalence of the micro-organisms concerned. For example, if staff caring for patients colonised with MRSA have a bacteriological skin swab taken, MRSA is frequently found on their skin. This does not mean that they are themselves colonised with MRSA; they are probably just transient carriers. This difficulty in detecting whether someone is a carrier or not is the reason why, when staff are being screened to eliminate MRSA carriage, they must always have swabs taken at the beginning of the staff member's span of duty and not the end. This will ensure that only staff who are colonised will be identified. Generally, transient micro-organisms do not survive on a person's skin for more than a few hours (Reybrouck, 1983). However, during this time they can be easily transmitted to other people or objects (Mackintosh and Hoffman, 1984). The way to stop this method of cross-infection is through handwashing (Figure 9.1).

Frequency of handwashing

In an ideal world, hands would always be washed before and after each patient contact to remove transient organisms. In hospital, this should be quite easily achieved as soap, handwash basins and paper hand towels are all generally within easy reach. This is not always the case in the

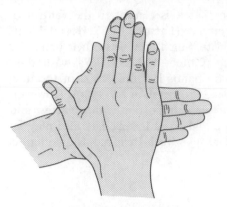

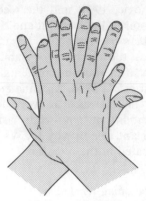

Wet hands and add solution.
Rub palms together.

Right palm over back of left hand and
left palm over back of right hand.

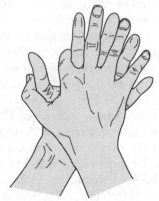

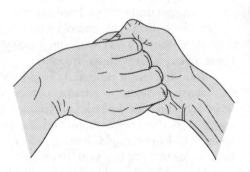

Palm to palm with
fingers interlaced

Rub backs of fingers with palm.

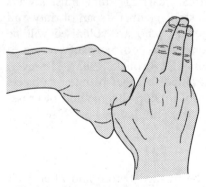

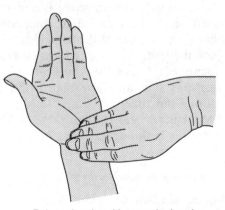

Wash each thumb by clasping and rotating
in the palm of the opposite hand.

Rub each wrist with opposite hand.
Rinse hands and dry.

community when HCWs are often in a situation where they may find it difficult or sometimes impossible to wash their hands. In these situations the use of an antiseptic handrub or handwipe, if the hands are physically dirty, is appropriate.

In the real world ideal practice is rarely achieved. To enable staff to understand when hands must be washed they must be educated to perform a risk assessment which should include:

- the degree of contact they are likely to have with patients or potentially contaminated objects such as bedpans and urinals;
- the susceptibility of patients they are caring for to infection such as patients in the intensive care unit or the very young;
- the procedure about to be performed such as a wound dressing or a lumbar puncture.

Handwashing standard

In health care setting, standards are being written so that health care practice can be monitored, evaluated and improved. Table 9.1 is an example of how a handwashing standard may look and how it could be monitored.

Methods of monitoring handwashing standard
Example questions for a questionnaire on hand cleansing prior to the introduction of standard, would include the following.

- How long does it take you to wash your hands at work?
- Lists of common procedures and questions as to whether hands should or should not be washed and what solutions should be used.

There should be weekly half-hourly monitoring of health care workers carried out by infection control practitioners, the audit department or infection control link nurses. Then there should be a questionnaire on hand cleansing after the introduction of the standard (Figure 9.1).

Categories of handwashing

Removal of transient flora
Fortunately, washing hands with soap or detergent for 15 to 20 seconds is normally effective enough to remove transient organisms (Ayliffe, Coates and Hoffman, 1993).

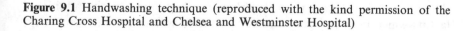

Figure 9.1 Handwashing technique (reproduced with the kind permission of the Charing Cross Hospital and Chelsea and Westminster Hospital)

Table 9.1 Handwashing standard

Care Group: all health care workers having patient contact
Standard statement: all health care workers will have clean hands prior to
carrying out invasive procedures

Structure	Process	Outcome
Handwash basins to be accessible and cleaned twice daily by domestic staff	Before each invasive procedure hands should be cleaned, either by: ● washing or	All staff to be aware of the importance of handwashing
Cleansing agent in dispenser regularly refilled: ● liquid soap for social/general handwashing ● alcoholic handrub for physically clean hands ● chlorhexidine solution prior to performing invasive procedures Nails to be kept short and any lesions on the hands or forearms should be covered with a waterproof plaster Paper handtowels available at all handwash basins Instructions on the correct method of handwashing available at all basins Waste bin for used paper hand towels at basins with pedal mechanism Handcream available in each ward/department	● alcoholic handrub can be used if physically clean *Handwashing* ● Wet hands thoroughly, removing wrist watches and rings if possible ● apply solution (3–5 ml): ● handwash for 15–30 seconds, (Figure 9.1) ● rinse hands thoroughly with running water ● dry hands thoroughly with a paper hand towel ● dispose of hand towel in pedal bin without touching lid ● repeat before each invasive procedure is performed *Handrub* Apply 3 ml of solution, rub as described above, until hands are dry	All staff to be aware of effective hand cleansing techniques

The 1985 CDC guideline (Garner and Favero, 1986) states that plain soap should be used for handwashing unless otherwise indicated. Until controlled clinical trials have proven that soap containing antimicrobial agents is more effective than plain soap, it should continue to be used (Larson, 1995). However, in health care there are certain additional factors which must be taken into consideration when choosing plain soap.

Plain soap should always be in the form of liquid soap not bar soap, as bar soap has been shown to support the growth of Gram-negative bacteria. Liquid soaps must also be dispensed in containers to eliminate the possibility for contamination, i.e. soap should not be continually topped up in a container, as this will allow bacterial growth. Plain soap and water should be used by most HCWs on a daily basis as they are an effective way of decontaminating hands (Huang *et al.*, 1994)

Removal of resident flora

Resident flora are considered permanent residents of the skin and are not readily removed by mechanical friction. Removal of resident skin flora is not usually necessary as they are not readily transferred to other people or surfaces and most are of low pathogenicity. However, some resident bacteria may cause infection if introduced during invasive procedures into normally sterile body sites, or to sites on particularly vulnerable individuals. In these circumstances antiseptic agents are necessary to kill or inhibit micro-organisms and reduce the level still further.

Antiseptic agents and alcohol handrubs

Antiseptic agents such as Hibiscrub and Betadine are soap solutions with an antiseptic added. They will remove the micro-organisms that normally live on the skin as well as the transient ones. There are three situations in which these have a role to play.

- Antiseptic soap is only necessary prior to invasive procedures, e.g. surgery, or before contact with patients who are very susceptible to infection, e.g. neonates or people in intensive care.
- Alcohol handrub solutions can be used as a quick method of removing micro-organisms from the hands if the hands are not already soiled.
- Alcohol handwipes may be used in the community when there is no access to soap or water.

Regardless of the solution, the removal of bacteria will only be effective if all parts of the hands are washed thoroughly (Taylor, 1978; Gidley, 1987). Any parts of the hands that are missed may be responsible for cross-infection. Most people when washing their hands tend to miss the thumb and forefinger of their dominant hand, and the webs of their fingers. This is why it is so important for staff to be shown how to wash their hands as well as told when to wash them.

It has been shown that, even when an antiseptic is used, there is a maximum level of reduction in bacterial counts that can be reached, regardless of frequency or intensity of handwashing (Lilly *et al.*, 1979). When choosing products, it is important to realise that alcohol-based preparations require less time to effect a maximum reduction than products containing chlorhexidine gluconate.

Detergent antiseptic solutions are designed to be used by operating theatre personnel a few times a day. When incorrectly used by staff such as routinely in clinical settings where staff frequently wash their hands they have been associated with skin damage and increased levels of bacteria on the hands. Therefore, they should only be used in the operating theatres. Some infection control practitioners (ICPs) have recommended their use in the control of nosocomial outbreaks. However, most ICPs agree that it is the reinforcement of handwashing which leads to outbreak control rather than the use of surgical handrubs.

Hand drying

A variety of methods are available for drying hands. Cloth towels have not been recommended for some considerable years in health care settings because of concerns regarding contamination (Robinton, 1968).

Hot air dryers which have, in recent years, become very common in public toilets and washrooms (Blackmore, 1989), due to the fact that they save money in waste collection and the supply of handtowels, are generally not recommended for health care premises (Ayliffe et al., 1993). Studies (Meers and Leong, 1989; Ansari et al., 1991) have shown that they do not reduce the amount of micro-organisms on the hands compared with paper hand towels and one study (Redway et al., 1994) has actually shown an increase in the flora. In practical terms hot air dryers are noisy, can serve only one person at a time and have a standard 30 second cycle, meaning that the user frequently walks away from the dryer with wet hands. People have been observed to simply walk away from the dryer without fully drying their hands, or wipe their hands on their clothes, a practice not to be encouraged in health care settings!

Finally, after hands have been washed and dried with paper hand towels, it is important that staff do not immediately recontaminate their hands by touching the waste bin lid with their hands when they throw the paper hand towel away. All bins in clinical areas should be foot operated.

Protective clothing, e.g. gloves, aprons and face protection

The wearing of protective clothing must be based on a risk assessment of the procedure to be performed. It is important to understand that the degree of risk of the procedure is not altered by any supposed infection that the individual has. It is the risk of the procedure itself which is being assessed.

Gloves, the most often used form of protective clothing, must always be worn by HCWs if there is a risk that they may come into contact with blood or body fluids during a procedure. Gloves should also be worn for procedures involving direct contact with non-intact skin or mucous membranes, for example mouth care and vaginal examinations. This is to protect both the member of staff as well as the patient. There is however considerable variability in the quality of gloves, with reports of leakage from both vinyl and latex gloves (DeGroot-Kosolchareon and Jones, 1989). A recent study has also shown that there was little benefit in double gloving with latex gloves (Korniewicz et al., 1994). Possible microbial contamination of hands and transmission of infection have been reported even when gloves are worn (Olsen et al., 1993). The wearing of gloves is often seen as obviating the need for handwashing (Lund et al., 1994). In the absence of definitive proof, current practice accepts that it does not. Hands must always be washed or an antiseptic handrub used after glove removal.

More widespread use of gloves has lead to increased reports of reactions to latex gloves. Dermatitis in HCWs may place patients at risk because handwashing will not decrease bacterial counts on damaged skin. HCWs with dermatitis may also be at increased risk of exposure to blood borne pathogens during skin contact with blood or body fluids as the normal protective barrier is not intact (Ridzon et al., 1997). Numerous solutions, from not wearing latex gloves to the use of emollients and hypoallergenic gloves have been suggested. It is also important to remember that some patients are themselves allergic to latex (Leynadier et al., 1989) and therefore an allergy history should always be obtained before latex gloves are used.

Single use gloves should never be washed/disinfected/resterilised and then reused as sterility cannot be guaranteed. It is also important to realise that HCWs do not only wear gloves to protect themselves from infection, they are also used to protect the client. Gloves must always be changed for each patient encounter, such as when taking blood (Vickers et al., 1994) as reusing gloves can lead to cross-infection with blood borne viruses (Heptonstall, 1993).

In the health care setting two main types of gloves are used, sterile and clean. Sterile gloves are far more expensive than clean and for this reason it is important that staff wear the right gloves. Sterile gloves need only be worn in certain procedures, for example when the hands are going to come into contact with normally sterile body areas, e.g. during surgical procedures and urinary catheter insertion. Clean gloves should be used at all other times including blood taking and giving normal intravenous drugs.

There is often confusion about glove usage during wound dressings. Clean gloves only need to be worn during wound dressings because of the way wounds heal. The process of wound healing is either by 'primary intention' or by 'secondary intention'. An example of a primary intention wound is a surgical wound. The wound edges are held together by mechanical aids, such as clips or sutures and the epithelial bridge (scab) forms within 48 hours of wound closure. Therefore there is no need, in most cases, for any form of dressing, and there is definitely no need for sterile gloves to be worn during dressing changes, as the wound is 'protected' by the scab. Secondary intention wounds, such as pressure sores or leg ulcers, are wounds which involve tissue loss. They are already colonised with bacteria and are therefore not sterile, so only clean gloves need be worn when changing dressings. Handwashing and the wearing of clean gloves should prevent the HCW from contaminating the wound when performing the dressing.

Handwashing and glove use are the two lynch pins of infection control and yet no data exists to determine which is the most important in preventing cross-infection. Glove use is expensive and with nosocomial infection rates already low (approximately 5% incidence) it is difficult to know whether 100% compliance with glove use, handwashing or both would actually significantly reduce the incidence. However, until there is some evidence to show which is the most effective, most ICPs will continue to advise that both are adopted.

For gloves to be used appropriately they must be readily available to staff in all areas; this is often easier to achieve in acute care settings than elsewhere. In the community, for example, there is still a general lack of understanding of the need for UICP as clients are often perceived as low infection risks, and therefore the purchase of gloves is often not seen as a high priority. However, as more and more community infection control nurses come into post this is gradually being challenged. In areas, such as residential homes, where residents are said to be 'in their own home' a practical compromise must be reached between infection control and their environment.

Nails, nail polish and artificial nails

The increasing use of artificial nails, particularly in the USA, has led to questions about whether HCWs should be allowed to use artificial nails when giving direct patient care. Reports have given different views on the risks of cross-infection with artificial nails. However, when the prosthetic nails were broken or had separated from the natural nails, high colony counts have been found (Pottinger et al., 1989).

Nail polish applied to natural nails does not appear to have any detrimental influence on the microbial load as long as the nails are short. Clear nail varnish is preferable to coloured, as colours make it difficult to view the long nails and notice any dirt. Keeping nails short is probably the most important factor as most flora on the hands is found under the fingernails. Also long nails can make donning gloves difficult, and may make gloves tear more easily. It has also been shown that the microbial contamination of hands in gloves is due to the flora under the nails being spread over the hands as the gloves are pulled on.

Jewellery

Bacterial counts are higher when rings are worn (Hoffman *et al.,* 1985; Gould, 1994). However many staff will not remove a wedding band, and rings have not been shown to interfere with the removal of bacteria during handwashing. Rings and nail jewellery can make donning gloves more difficult and may cause gloves to tear readily, and they may also cause injury to patients when being physically lifted or turned.

Hand lotions

Lotions are often recommended to ease the dryness associated with frequent hand washing. However it is important that hand lotion in communal pots is avoided as contamination has been shown to occur and can be a source of cross-infection (Morse and Schonbeck, 1968).

Broken skin

Damaged skin contains higher numbers of micro-organisms. Cuts and abrasions should be covered with a waterproof dressing, not one that is just water resistant, as these will protect the cut/abrasion and enable the HCWs to continue to wash their hands. They should also wear gloves whenever a risk assessment suggests possible contamination.

Aprons and water repellent and resistant gowns

Clean disposable plastic aprons should be worn whenever there is a risk of contamination of clothing with blood or body fluid. There has been frequent debate as to whether plastic aprons or cotton gowns should be used when caring for patients. The front of the body is exposed most frequently to direct contact with the patient and therefore plastic aprons are the most appropriate form of protective clothing to be worn the majority of the time. Whenever the HCW is going to be exposed to fluid, plastic aprons must be worn, e.g. during bed baths, removing bedpans and when clearing up body fluids as in these situations a cotton gown is totally inappropriate. Disposable plastic aprons should be available in all clinical areas, and the home. Economically, it costs far more to launder a cotton balloon cloth gown than to provide clean disposable plastic aprons for staff to wear on a regular basis.

There are some procedures during which the risk of the HCW coming into contact with blood and body fluid, notably during some surgical interventions or in A and E departments, is much higher. In such circumstances the HCW should have access to water repellent gowns. In the past staff have often worn a plastic apron under a normal cotton gown.

This does not protect the forearms or upper arms and shoulders. There are many different makes of water repellent gowns available on the market – some single use disposable and other reusable ones which are made of a special material or treated cotton. However, they are expensive, but, despite the cost, many operating departments in the UK recommend their use for all procedures where there is a risk to the HCW of exposure to blood or body fluid. Most commercial laundries provide these gowns and, as more and more provider units rent their linen and theatre wear from commercial laundries, they are becoming more accessible to HCWs.

Eye and face protection

Masks were first worn in the operating theatre with the intention of protecting the patient from organisms found in the upper respiratory tract of the HCW. However, it is now realised that most of the bacteria dispersed by talking and sneezing from a healthy member of staff is in fact harmless to wounds (Ayliffe *et al.*, 1992). Masks are therefore not necessary in most procedures to protect the patient.

The emphasis today is on wearing masks to protect the HCW and it is accepted that the scrub team for an operation should wear masks to protect their faces from splashes of blood or body fluids. Staff have acquired a blood borne virus following occupational exposure from blood splashes to the face (Heptonstall *et al.*, 1993).

The re-emergence of tuberculosis and multi-drug resistant tuberculosis (MDRTB) has resulted in infection control practitioners re-evaluating the use of masks in hospitals. Traditionally, it was agreed that the efficacy of surgical face masks was not proven, and in the USA the use of disposable particulate respirators was advocated when HCWs were caring for people with tuberculosis. Particulate respirators include dust-mist (DM), dust-fume-mist (DFM) or high-efficiency particulate air (HEPA) filter respirators. In some units in the UK, when HIV positive clients with tuberculosis are receiving care, particulate respirators are now being used. However it is important to remember that masks should not be used alone when dealing with MDRTB; single rooms should be used which have a lower or negative air pressure compared with the surrounding area, vented to the outside atmosphere.

Face protection should be available and worn by staff whenever there is a risk of blood splashes to the face. This will occur not just in the operating room, but also in the labour wards, and dialysis and broncho-scopy units. The latest designs of glasses/goggles available are much more comfortable to wear and most importantly are easy to see out of. Under COSHH, eye protection should also be worn when staff are preparing and using certain drugs and when handling some chemicals. Unfortunately many staff are still exposed to unnecessary risk because such protective clothing is not readily available.

Safe handling and disposal of sharps

The dangers of using sharps (any item which can penetrate the skin) and ways to reduce the risks associated with their use have been extensively highlighted (Heptonstall *et al.*, 1993; Jagger *et al.*, 1990; Eisenstein and Smith, 1992; Mercier, 1994) Injuries from sharps are the major way in which a HCW occupationally acquires a blood borne virus. However, despite all the available evidence, staff continue to sustain sharps injuries and regrettably many are due to bad practice, and therefore avoidable (Mercier, 1994). The most effective way to prevent sharps injuries is to monitor exposures, report the results to the health care workers, and use appropriate interventions to address the risk (Lynch *et al.*, 1992). Although this is beginning to happen in hospitals and health centres, in the community (particularly in GP and dental surgeries) there is often no mechanism for reporting injuries and therefore no information on which to base rational intervention strategies.

All sharps must always be used in as safe a manner as possible by the HCW. It has been shown (Gerberding, 1991) that knowing that someone has a blood borne virus does not make the HCW less likely to sustain a sharps injury. This includes the disposal of the needles, blade or other sharp instruments, which should be placed directly into a rigid sharps container complying to United Nations 3291 (formerly BS7320; BSI, 1990).

Resheathing needles, bending needles

Needles must never be bent and should not be resheathed unless absolutely necessary and if they are resheathed then a one handed scoop method should be used, i.e. the sheath is placed on a surface and the needle inserted using one hand only. Since the sheath is not held at all the risk of a needlestick injury is eliminated.

Disposal of sharps

All sharps must be disposed of safely and correctly immediately after use. The method of disposal of needles used by diabetics differs across the country. In some areas diabetics are given sharps bins which are collected for incineration. In other places this does not happen. If diabetics are not provided with sharps bins and a collection service they should use needle clippers which will make the needle safe, and can store up to 200 needles. The needle clippers are disposed of as household waste.

Types of sharps which cause injury

Care should always be taken when using the types of sharps which cause most injuries (i.e. needles, scalpels and suture needles).

Sharps containers

All sharps bins must comply with UN 3291, be accessible but in a safe position, and disposed of by incineration when 3/4 full. As with all clinical waste, it is good practice for sharps bins to be labelled with their point of origin before being sent for incineration.

Staff education

People tend to resist recommendations made by others. Educational initiatives around the prevention of sharps injuries by the occupational health and/or infection control teams will therefore have a much greater chance of success if the relevant HCWs are actively involved from the start.

The risk to HCWs from sharps injuries is that they will acquire a blood borne virus, e.g. HIV, hepatitis B or hepatitis C. The risk of acquiring hepatitis B following an inoculation sharps injury involving blood from a hepatitis B carrier is approximately 1 in 3; hepatitis C, approximately 1 in 10; and HIV approximately 1 in 300.

Treatment of sharps injuries

Accidents with blood and body fluids occur both in the hospital and the community. Any exposure to blood or body fluids from a sharps injury, bite, or from splashing to the eyes, mouth or non-intact skin must always be treated because of the risk of infection (Figure 9.2). Such injuries often give rise to a great deal of anxiety in the person sustaining the injury. Because of this the first consideration should be prevention of the injury through always following safe written procedures, e.g. during venepuncture and using safe evaluated equipment. When an accident has occurred, the emphasis should be on secondary prevention of infection with a blood borne virus. For this reason, since 1994, all HCWs who perform invasive procedures have been required to have the HBV vaccination. This is to protect the HCW and their clients.

Action following sharps injury or exposure to blood/body fluids

In the case of any of the following occurring:

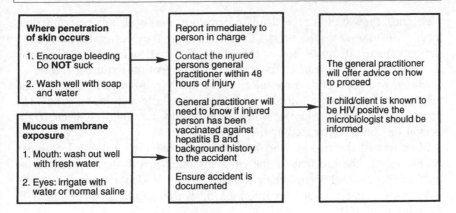

Figure 9.2 Accidental exposure to blood or sharp object contaminated with blood/ needle stick injury

- an injury from a used needle or sharp instrument;
- splashing into the face, especially the mouth and eyes;
- spillage on to open skin cuts, including areas affected by eczema;
- contamination of the HCW by a patient/client's blood or body fluid to such an extent that a change of clothing is necessary. Immediate action should be taken.

Immediate action following the incident

- If it is a small wound, encourage bleeding by squeezing area, do not suck.
- Wash area thoroughly with soap and running water.
- If the eyes/mouth are involved irrigate with sterile saline or tap water for 1–2 minutes.
- Inform the manager and complete an incident form.
- Report to occupational health/A and E immediately. Staff working in general practice should seek advice from the general practitioner, or if not possible go to the nearest A and E department.

Spillages of blood or body fluids onto intact skin need to be washed off immediately and no further action is required. If a member of staff sustains a sharps injury they need to implement immediate first aid (Figure 9.2) and complete an accident/incident form and take it with them to occupational health/A and E. This is so that the reasons for injuries within the area can be analysed, and it is also legal documentation of the incident. If a GP is dealing with an injury to a member of their staff they should record all information and seek advice from their local consultant virologist(s). On attending the occupational health department or, if out of hours, the A and E department, staff will receive a confidential assessment of the degree of intervention required, if any.

Many provider units now offer a 24 hour pre-recorded confidential advice line on sharps injuries and the immediate action to take. The provider unit's local sharps injury policy must be followed even if the person has been vaccinated against hepatitis B.

Members of the public, who have been injured with a discarded sharp, should report the incident to the environmental health department of the local authority and attend their nearest A and E department. The main risks from a sharps injury involving blood is that of acquiring hepatitis B, hepatitis C or HIV.

If the source of the injury is known, members of staff will normally collect all the details. This means that, providing consent is gained from the patient, blood can be taken from the source to establish the risks. If the risk of an infection with a blood borne virus is confirmed, one or more of the following guidelines should be implemented.

Guidelines following infection fron a blood borne virus

Hepatitis B

Hepatitis B is a blood borne and sexually transmitted virus. Depending on the age when infection occurs, a chronic carrier state occurs in 10–50% of persons infected. Hepatitis B surface antigen was previously known as Australian antigen. Immunisation is not effective in approximately 5% of the population, but if seroconversion occurs, the chronic carrier state is prevented even though super infection may occur. Prevalence varies from country to country. The background level in the UK is one per 1 000 population rising to 15–20% in some ethnic minority groups. Acute infection is associated with a mortality of 1% and significant morbidity. The chronic carrier status is the commonest cause of liver cancer. The risk of infection is from blood, blood products and peritoneal dialysis fluid from a person who is hepatitis B surface antigen (HBsAg) positive. Other body fluids only present a risk when they are blood stained.

The degree of exposure is assessed. If the exposure risk is considered low, such as blood on to intact skin, no further action will be taken. The risk is considered high when the following occurs:

- percutaneous inoculation, such as a sharps injury or a human bite which punctures the skin;
- contamination of non-intact skin, such as fresh cuts less than 24 hours old, or eczema/psoriasis;

- splashing to the eyes or mouth;
- unprotected sexual intercourse.

In these situations the following will be done.

- If the identity of the source is known, consent to a blood test for HBV markers may be requested, and people should be given an explanation of the reason for the tests. If the result is negative no further action is necessary. However, if the person sustaining the injury has not had an immunisation course for hepatitis B one should be commenced.
- When the identity of the source is unknown or the person refuses consent, an assessment of probable risk should be undertaken, in accordance with national guidance (Hepatitis subcommittee; PHLS, 1992).
- If the source is positive, immunisation should be provided (Table 9.2) dependent on an individual's current immune status. People who have had such injuries need to be counselled with regard to their sex lives and need to be followed up. Pregnancy is not a contraindication to immunisation following a potential exposure.

Hepatitis C

Hepatitis C is now known to be one of the causes of non-A, non-B hepatitis. As it has only been recognised recently the understanding of the epidemiology is incomplete. It is known to be a blood borne virus with similar routes of transmission to hepatitis B. However the risk of transmission associated with sexual exposure remains unclear.

Most people infected with HCV are asymptomatic. Irrespective of the clinical symptoms at the time of infection, HCV can persist and cause liver damage 20–30 years later. If a HCW has an inoculation injury and the source is known to have hepatitis C antibodies there is a risk they may acquire hepatitis C. There is no vaccine: the only treatment available is interferon.

Following an injury, blood should be taken if possible from the source together with baseline bloods from the HCW who sustained the injury. Further samples can then be taken at three and six months for liver function tests and HCV antibodies.

HIV

HIV is the cause of AIDS. Following infection with the virus, seroconversion normally occurs six to ten weeks later and is associated in 10% of cases with a clinical sero-conversion syndrome. After a latent period of 12 to 15 years during which time there is a progressive loss of CD4 lymphocytes the person becomes increasingly susceptible to AIDS indicator diseases, such as *Pneumocystis carinii* pneumonia (PCP), tuber-

Table 9.2 HBV prophylaxis for reported exposure incidents[a]

HBV status of person exposed	Significant exposure			Non-significant exposure	
	positive source	HBsAg unknown source	negative source	HBsAg continued risk	no further risk
< dose HB vaccine pre-exposure	Accelerated course of HB vacc* HBIG × 1	Accelerated course of HB vaccine*	Initiate course of HB vaccine	Initiate course of HB vaccine	No HBV prophylaxis Reassure
> 2 doses HB vaccine pre-exposure (anti-HBs unknown)	One dose of HB vaccine followed by 2nd dose 1 month later	One dose of HB vaccine	Finish course of HB vaccine	Finish course HB vaccine	No HBV prophylaxis Reassure
Known responder to HB vaccine (anti-HBs > 10miU/ml)	Booster dose of HB vaccine	Consider booster dose of HB vacc	Consider booster dose of HB vacc	Consider booster dose of HB vacc	No HBV prophylaxis Reassure
Known nonresponder to HB vaccine (anti-HBs < 10miU/ml 2–4 months post vaccination)	HBIG × 1 Consider booster dose of HB vacc	HBIG × 1 Consider booster dose of HB vacc	No HBIG Consider booster dose of HB vacc	No HBIG Consider booster dose of HB vacc	No HBV prophylaxis Reassure

[a] Derived from *CDR* (1992) **2**, Review No. 9, R99.
* An accelerated course of vaccine consists of doses spaced at 0, 1 and 2 months. A booster is given at 12 months to those at continuing risk of exposure to HBV.

culosis and Kaposi's sarcoma. Currently, there is no vaccine and no treatment which significantly alters the clinical course of the disease, although prophylactic antibiotics, for example pentamidine for PCP, may reduce the incidence of inter-current disease.

HIV has been transmitted to HCWs following inoculation injuries with HIV positive blood or contamination of damaged skin with blood, (Heptonstall *et al.*, 1993). As with all such incidents, staff must attend the occupational health department or if out of hours, the A and E department. The HIV risk will be assessed as for HBV.

In most infections the HIV status of the source will be unknown. If there is a need to know, it is essential that the patient is offered counselling by a professional counsellor as the patient must give their consent before any testing is performed. Following injury zidovudine is often recommended in an attempt to eliminate HIV. Evidence to date indicates that in most cases this is unsuccessful (Heptonstall *et al.*, 1993).

Creutzfeldt-Jakob disease

Creutzfeldt-Jakob disease (CJD) is one of the causes of spongiform encephalopathy. Most of the reports of cross-infection with CJD have been associated with neurosurgery or corneal transplant. However, there is also concern that it may be related to the consumption of beef infected with bovine spongiform encephalitis (BSE). In health care, if UICPs are followed at all times there should rarely be any extra precautions to be taken. However, if surgery is going to be performed on a patient with suspected CJD, certain procedures must be followed (DoH, 1992; HSAC, 1991). There should be minimal people in the operating theatre, and all equipment should be single-use disposable. If this is not possible used instruments usually need to be incinerated.

If an inoculation injury occurs with an object contaminated with cerebrospinal fluid or any part of the central nervous system of a patient known to have CJD, there may be a risk of transmission, although this is presently unknown. No prophylactic measures are available and no treatment. Advice should be sought from a consultant neurologist.

Viral haemorrhagic fevers

Viral haemorrhagic fevers (VHFs) include infections caused by the Lassa and Ebola viruses. Transmission is by blood and body fluids, and there have been cases when HCWs have acquired the diseases. Any HCW who has contact with a patient with a VHF will routinely have their temperature recorded for 21 days. If they develop a fever over 38°C they will be admitted to an infectious diseases unit.

If a HCW sustains an inoculation injury from a patient with suspected

VHF the diagnosis will need to be confirmed. Lassa Fever can be treated, but advice must be sought from the local infectious diseases unit and the PHLS.

Spillages

In health care, clearing up spillages of blood or body fluids may expose the HCW to pathogens. When dealing with any spills it is essential to wear the appropriate protective clothing, which in all cases will be clean gloves and, dependent on the amount of spill, may include a plastic apron. The HCW must have a clinical waste (yellow) bag available to put the waste in (Figure 9.3). All spills should be dealt with as quickly as possible. The HCW discovering the spill will generally be the person who should clear it up. Most provider units, clinics, etc. have policies for who clears up spills in communal areas. The most dangerous spills are those of blood or body fluid visibly stained with blood. In some areas, such as pathology departments, where glass tubes are used there may be the

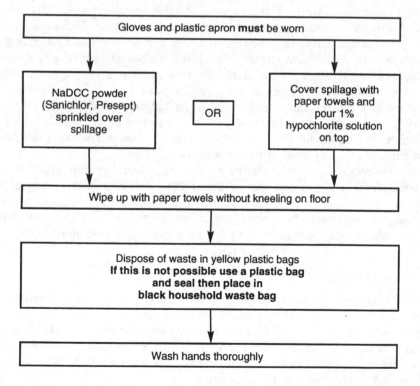

Figure 9.3 Blood spillage

additional hazard of sharps in the spill. To deal with these there are now available plastic disposable 'dustpans' and a plastic disposable shovel, which enables the sharps to be safely cleared away once they have been decontaminated with chlorine granules and left for an appropriate length of time. Chlorine granules (Chapter 10) have the advantage of containing the spill rather than adding to it, however if they are not available, the area may be covered with disposable hand towels and a bleach solution poured on top. Then, wearing gloves and apron, the granules should be removed with disposable wipes, discarded into a yellow bag to be sent for incineration and the area washed over with neutral detergent (washing up liquid) and water. In the home, bleach (hypochlorite) can be used. However, bleach is corrosive to certain metals and will stain fabrics and carpets. Therefore, it is generally preferable to soak the spill up using disposable cloths or, if not available, newspaper and to clean the area with detergent and water.

Bleach solutions should not be used on urine spills as the acid in the urine reacts with the hypochlorite to release toxic chlorine gas. Urine spills should be absorbed by using disposable paper towels/wipes/ newspaper and wiped over with neutral detergent and water.

Spillage of vaccines

Vaccine spillages must be dealt with as blood and body fluid spills. The disinfectant of choice is hypochlorite. Any unused or out of date vaccines must be disposed of as special waste.

Excreta

Excreta should be discarded directly into the bedpan washer/macerator or toilet. If this is not possible, for example if someone is incontinent of faeces in bed, excreta must be placed in a yellow bag and sent for incineration. In the home setting disposable nappies and incontinent wipes can be placed into normal household waste and sent for landfill.

Environment factors

The environment in which someone is treated has a very important association with the risk of the person acquiring an infection and the type of infection.

Hospitals

As already outlined (Chapter 1), hospitals have generally been associated with death since time immemorial. Not just death from infection but from accidents. Florence Nightingale said that hospitals should do the sick no harm (*Notes on Nursing*), and this is something we should still be striving for today.

It is generally accepted that a wide variety of pathogenic micro-organisms, including some strains resistant to many antibiotics are to be found in the hospital setting. Nosocomial or hospital acquired infection (HAI) is defined as any infection which the person develops as a result of treatment in a hospital (including day surgery). Nosocomial infection is difficult to identify following day surgery. With a length of stay of less than 24 hours, it is difficult to ascertain the precise time of infection, and patients are rarely followed up in the community after discharge. There has been little work done on the human and financial cost of nosocomial infections in the UK. The major source of data comes from the USA and relates to hospital inpatient data for the 1970s and early 1980s. This USA Study on the Efficacy of Nosocomial Infection Control (SENIC) (Haley *et al.*, 1985) showed that between 5 and 6% of patients admitted to USA hospitals acquired an infection. This obviously has huge cost implications. The SENIC study also showed that a properly conducted programme of surveillance and control prevented 32% of cases of HAI. This has to date not been evaluated in the UK. These data are now very old and are derived from a country with a very different health care system to the UK. It is therefore unwise to extrapolate directly from this study and to apply its recommendations to the UK in the late 1990s. However, it does unfortu-nately remain the only data available, and until further work is done in the UK the true cost and most effective way of preventing nosocomial infections will not be known.

It is known that different specialties are associated with different infection risks. Operating theatres, for example, have some of the most stringent guidance regarding building and maintenance, in recogni-tion of the susceptibility of people undergoing major invasive procedures. Many HAIs are caused by opportunistic pathogens introduced into susceptible sites by invasive procedures such as surgical joint replace-ments.

There has been publicity in the press regarding the general lack of cleanliness in hospitals and whether this is an infection risk. While more and more new hospitals are being built in the UK, a great many patients are still being cared for in out-of-date buildings with poor handwashing facilities and inadequate space to house much of the present day technology. It is probably this lack of space, the inadequate numbers of single rooms and poor or inaccessible handwashing facilities that increases the infection risk. Although in some areas, particularly toilets and the operating departments, lack of cleaning may create a serious infection risk.

The community

The infections that people acquire in their own homes are very different from those associated with hospital. This is mainly because of the minor nature of the procedures undertaken in the community, and because drug resistant bacteria are also less common, so that when infections do occur they are easily treated.

However, times are changing and patients are being discharged home from hospital earlier. Many infections identified in the community may be the result of an infection originally acquired in the hospital, but no signs were visible while the person was an inpatient. Nevertheless the trend for the community is for increasingly susceptible patients to be treated in their home environment, this will inevitably lead to people in the community acquiring more difficult-to-treat infections.

Isolation precautions

In hospitals, patients may be isolated from other patients and staff either because their condition renders them at risk of infection from others, (the term usually used is 'protective isolation'), or because they themselves are potentially a source of infection. This is often referred to as 'barrier nursing' or being placed in 'source isolation'. This second form of isolation is based on the old tradition of keeping people with infection away from others who are not infected. Many of the terms used create the impression of locking the patient away, which in effect is what did happen a 100 years ago in fever hospitals. Research has been carried out into the effect of isolation on patients in protective isolation (Collins *et al.*, 1989), but little work has been carried out on patients placed in 'source isolation' (Knowles, 1993). Patients in protective isolation are much more involved in the decision to be isolated, having often had time to prepare for the experience, than those who are isolated because they have a communicable disease.

In the community, it could be said that people with infections staying at home and not going to work or school are, in a way, isolating themselves.

If UICPs were followed at all times and if all patients were cared for in single rooms there would rarely be a need to isolate patients in hospital. Unfortunately, this is not so and throughout the hospitals in the UK various isolation methods have been established. Isolation is often deemed necessary in hospital as patients with infectious diseases can present a potential source of disease to staff and patients, though the reason for isolation and the effect it may have on the patient, their family and friends must always be taken into consideration. There may be occasions, when the patient is confused or distressed when they should not be isolated as it would be detrimental to their wellbeing. Another reason why patients are frequently not isolated in hospital is that the facilities for isolation are not available. This is often the case in older hospitals that do not have enough side rooms, and areas like the intensive care or high dependency units where again there may not be enough side rooms, or staff to care for them. In these situations the ICT must take an active part in discussing the care of the patient and how to prevent the spread of infection.

While the need for additional precautions being taken with some communicable diseases, such as properly evaluated masks being worn by HCWs caring for clients with potentially multi-drug resistant tuberculosis is generally accepted, the exact value of isolating patients has never been fully researched. Many aspects of nursing are still based on tradition rather than research, and isolation precautions can be included in this group. Isolation is also still generally seen as part of nursing not medicine in general, as can be seen in the terms 'isolation or barrier nursing'. With the introduction of UICP there should very rarely be a need to isolate people in the hospital setting.

DIFFERENT ISOLATION PROCEDURES

Historically, in the past 20 years there have been two systems for isolation procedures.

Disease specific

Many current isolation procedures are based on following a set of guidelines once a diagnosis has been made. An example of this would be salmonella gastroenteritis, an infection spread through faecal contact. Advocates of disease specific isolation precautions believe that, by only following precautions when you know someone is infectious, resources are only used when they are needed, thereby saving time and money. This is difficult to justify as someone does not suddenly become infectious, or more infectious once an infectious organism has been isolated. Often people are infectious for several days before the illness becomes apparent and a causative organism is identified only later. It is generally accepted that everyone may potentially be carrying a blood borne pathogen, so it should be accepted that anyone can carry any pathogen without necessarily showing any signs or symptoms of an infectious disease, or even a diagnosis ever being made. If gloves are always worn and hands washed after a HCW has contact with excreta, there should only very rarely be a need to place a patient with a known enteric infection into a side room.

Categories of isolation

This system puts groups of diseases into different categories. A strict category would be used for a disease such as viral haemorrhagic fevers, which would not normally be seen outside of an infectious diseases unit. A respiratory category would be used for TB and chickenpox, wound and skin category for any infected or colonised wounds and enteric category for gastrointestinal illnesses. This group of four different types of isolation requires the HCW to be constantly vigilant as to which precautions they should be following. It is very prescriptive and in certain cases, can lead to a patient being in more than one category. For example, in a patient with a small round structured virus, a symptom of which is diarrhoea but which can be spread by people inhaling and ingesting vomit. While accepting that isolation precautions do have a role to play, it is important to evaluate them. One of the areas where isolating patients has become the accepted basis of control is MRSA (Figure 9.4) and yet, despite this emphasis on single room isolation, the numbers of patients with MRSA in the 1980s and 1990s has continuously increased. Barrier nursing in this context is obviously not working.

In most general hospitals there will need to be three categories of isolation; strict, standard and protective.

Strict isolation

In a general hospital, strict isolation would only ever be used in the A and E department if someone comes in who is suspected of having a viral haemorrhagic fever (VHF). Anyone suspected of having one of these diseases, such as Lassa fever or Ebola fever is deemed highly infectious and must be transferred immediately to one of the designated infectious diseases units around the country. Such patients will be cared for in a plastic Trexlor isolator which has negative air pressure and air locks. Staff who have contact with any such patients are monitored for 21 days.

Standard isolation

Standard isolation is the most common method of isolating all patients with the common infections which may be spread in the hospital. It is vitally important that staff understand when patients should be placed in isolation and when they should come out. In most hospitals, standard isolation means being placed in a single room. For some infections there is a logic behind this, e.g. airborne infections such as chickenpox and TB, but generally, compliance with the basic principle of infection control, i.e. handwashing, is the most effective component of isolation. Some ICPs believe that compliance with handwashing is better observed

Day 1   **Date:**

Patient name: _____   Hospital no: _____

		N/A	Signature
Medical	Prescribe for 5 days:		
	• Mupiricin nasal spray 3 times a day		
	• Mupiricin to wound edges twice a day		
	• Ster-Zac powder to groin and axilla		
	• Chlorhexidine 0.4% wash		
	Ring infection control doctor for antibiotics advice		
Nursing	Give patient isolation booklet and give explanation		
	Standard isolation procedure commenced (as infection control guidelines)		
	Place red standard isolation notice on door		
	Place aprons, gloves, alcohol hand rub outside room		
	All staff aware of:		
	Washing hands with chlorhexidine 0.4% when leaving room, and apply handrub		
	Domestic supervisor informed		
	Dip swabs in medium before swabbing nose, throat, groin, axilla and any wounds		
	Take CSU if patient has indwelling catheter		
	Send swabs to laboratory		
Domestic staff	Ensure room has: 1 green mop, 1 green bucket, green cloths		
Infection control team	Ensure patient is in standard isolation		
	Check MRSA antibiotic sensitivities		
	Check patient's contacts		
	Contact screening		
	MRSA sticker on notes		
	PAS informed		
Pharmacy			

Figure 9.4 Integrated care pathway: MRSA

(Affix patient label if available)

Patient's name: _____

Medical record No: _____

Sex: _____

Diagnosis: _____

Date of birth: _____

Consultant: _____

Ward: _____

Date MRSA detected: / /

Date MRSA clear: / /

Abbreviations on pathway

ICP	Integrated care pathway	PAS	Patient administrative system
MRSA	Methicillin resistant *Staphylococcus aureus*	CSU	Catheter specimen of urine

---

Notes for completing the ICP

Medical staff – please sign actions in bold type   *All other staff – please sign actions in italic type*

The person taking responsibility for an action being completed should sign the pathway (in full).

In the box next to the action, please put in a:

✓   if action is completed and sign.

✗   if action is not completed and sign. Please indicate the reason for the variance and the action taken on the variance sheet.

N/A   if action is not applicable and sign.

An ICP is not a rigid protocol and you must use your professional judgement to decide if following the pathway is appropriate.

---

if patients are in single rooms. The correct use of protective clothing is also vital.

Many HCWs feel that because a patient is in isolation they need to put on protective clothing each time they enter the room. This is not true; the same risk assessment procedure used for all UICPs should be put into practice when caring for someone in isolation. Staff may also cause unnecessary anxiety to the patient's family and friends by insisting that they wear protective clothing, when there is no evidence that the wearing of protective clothing by relatives has any role at all to play in preventing cross-infection. Staff wear protective clothing because they have contact with other patients; this is very rarely the case with relatives. It is, however, good practice for visitors to wash their hands on leaving the patient's room. In some cases, such as when a patient has chickenpox, it is advisable for visitors to be told of the potential for spread. Another infection, tuberculosis, is now raising some questions. Any visitors who have seen the patient in the preceding few weeks will have already had contact with the disease. Therefore restricting visiting is rarely necessary and also frequently unenforceable.

It is the role of the ICT through their input on the staff induction programmes and in service training to ensure that all staff understand why and when patients should be isolated and which type of protective clothing should be worn. It is vitally important that patients and their families and friends are aware of the reasons for isolation. Placing a patient in isolation may cause the patient stress and anxiety. Often, they do not understand why they have been isolated, and no one explains the reasons to their family and friends. Most ICTs now have information leaflets which give basic information about why a patient is being isolated and the name and contact numbers of the ICTs. These should be readily available on each ward so that as soon as a patient is isolated they are given easy to read, basic information, including a section for questions and reasons for isolation in a single room. They should be in the languages used by people who use the service, and an adapted leaflet for children and their parents/guardians should be available in paediatric areas. However, this leaflet should not detract from the important role of the ICT in visiting all patients in isolation and discussing any problems with them. To do this there has to be good communication between the ward/department staff and the ICT so that the ICT are informed of isolated patients. It is vitally important that staff follow up negative results and are as quick to take people out of isolation as to put them in.

Protective isolation

Another form of isolation is that of protective isolation which is used for people who are immunocompromised, such as a patient undergoing a bone marrow transplant. In this situation, patients are cared for in a single room, and the only real restriction is that staff, who have colds or are in any way feeling unwell, are not allowed to enter.

SUMMARY OF UICPs

Good practice in the health care environment should reduce the spread of infection, and includes:

Table 9.3 UICPs for all staff and clients

Potential pathogens will not spread easily from staff to client and client to staff
Recognising that used sharps are a hazard and must be disposed of safely
Ongoing commitment by employees to provide induction and inservice training
Taking the trouble to use protective clothing provided correctly
Ensuring that all cuts and abrasions on hands and arms are covered prior to starting work
Careful attention to handwashing technique
Time taken to ensure all waste, including soiled linen is disposed of safely
Infection control policies and guidelines available for all staff to read
Observance of the law which underpins good practice
Never being judgemental, anyone can carry infection.

- handwashing technique;
- safe handling and disposal of sharps, and good practice when dealing with injuries;
- correct use of protective clothing;
- appropriate isolation precautions.

For all staff and clients universal infection control precautions mean 'protection' (Table 9.3).

REFERENCES

Ansari, S.A., Springthorpe, V.S., Sattar, S.A., *et al.* (1991a) Comparison of cloth, paper and warm air drying in eliminating viruses and bacteria from washed hands. *American Journal of Infection Control*, **19**, 243–49.

Ansari, S.A., Springthorpe, V.S., Sattar, S.A., *et al.* (1991b) Potential role of hands in the spread of respiratory viral infections: studies with human parainfluenza virus 3 and rhinovirus 14. *Journal of Clinical Microbiology*, **29**, 2115–19.

Ayliffe, G.A.J., Lowbury, E.J.L., Geddes, A.M. and Williams, J.D. (1992) *Control of Hospital Infection. A practical handbook*, 3rd edn, Chapman & Hall Medical, London.

Ayliffe, G.A.J., Coates, D. and Hoffman, P.N. (1993) *Chemical Disinfection in Hospitals*, 2nd edn, Blackmore Press, Shaftesbury.

Blackmore, M.A. (1989) A comparison of hand drying methods. *Catering and Health*, **1**, 189–98.

Broughall, J.M., Marshman, C., Jackson, B. and Bird, P. (1984) An automatic monitoring system for measuring handwashing frequency in hospital wards. *Journal of Hospital Infection*, **5**, 447–53.

BSI (1990) BS 7320 British Standards Specifications for Sharps Containers, British Standards Institute, London.

Casewell, M. and Phillips, I. (1977) Hands as a route of transmission for *Klebsiella* spp. *British Medical Journal*, **ii**, 1315–17.

Centres for Disease Control (CDC) (1987) Recommendations for prevention of transmission of HIV transmission in health-care settings. *MMWR*, **36** (supp. no. 2S).

Collins, C., Upright, C. and Alekish, J. (1989) Reverse isolation: what patients perceive. *Oncological Nursing Forum*, **16**, (5), 675–79.

The Control of Substances Hazardous to Health (COSHH) Regulations (1994) SI:3246. *Tech. Rep.*

DeGroot–Kosolchareon, J. and Jones, J.M. (1989) Permeability of latex and vinyl gloves to water and blood. *American Journal of Infection Control*, **17**, 196–201.

Department of Health (1992) Neuro and ophthalmic surgery procedures on patients with or suspected to have, or at risk of developing, Creutzfeldt-Jakob disease (CJD) or Gerstmann-Straussler-Scheinker Syndrome (GSS) PL(92)CO/4. *Tech. Rep.*

Eisenstein, H.C. and Smith, D.A. (1992) Epidemiology of reported sharps injuries in a tertiary care hospital. *Journal of Hospital Infection*, **20**, 271–80.

Garner, J.S. and Simmons, B.P. (1983) Guideline for isolation precautions in hospitals. *Infection Control*, **4**, 245–325.

Garner, J.S. and Favero, M.S. (1989) CDC guideline for handwashing and hospital environmental control. *Infection Control*, **7**, 231–35.

General Dental Council (GDC) (1993) *Professional conduct and fitness to practice*, GDC, London.

Gerberding, J.L. (1991) Does knowledge of human immunodeficiency disease decrease the frequency of occupational exposure to blood? *American Journal of Medicine*, **91**, suppl. 3B, 312–19.

Gidley, C. (1987) Now, wash your hands! *Nursing Times*, **83**, (29), 40–2.

Gould, D. (1995) Nurses' hand decontamination practice; results of a local study. *Journal of Hospital Infection*, **28**, 15–30.

Haley, R.W., Culver, D.H. and White, J.W., *et al.* (1985) The efficacy of infection surveillance and control programs in preventing nosocomial infections in US hospitals (SENIC) Study. *American Journal of Epidemiology*, **121**, 182–205.

Health and Safety Executive (1988) *Control of Substances Hazardous to Health Regulations (1988)*, HMSO, London.

Health Services Advisory Committee (1991) *Safe Working and the Prevention of Infection in the Mortuary and Post-mortem Room*, HMSO, London.

Heptonstall, J., Gill, O.N., Porter, K., *et al.* (1993) Health care workers and HIV: surveillance of occupationally acquired infection in the United Kingdom. *CDR Review*, **3**, (11), R147–R153.

Hoffman, P.N., Cooke, E.M., McCarville, M.R. *et al.* (1985) Micro-organisms isolated from skin under wedding rings worn by hospital staff. *British Medical Journal*, **290**, 206–7.

Huang, Y., Oie, S. and Kamiya, A. (1994) Comparative effectiveness of hand-cleansing agents for removing methicillin-resistant *Staphylococcus aureus* from experimentally contaminated fingertips. *AJIC*, **22**, (4), 224–27.

Jagger, J., Hunt, J. and Pearson, R.D. (1990) Sharp object injuries in the hospital: causes and strategies for prevention. *American Journal of Infection Control*, **18**, (4), 227–31.

Knowles, H.E. (1993) The experience of infectious patients in isolation. *Nursing Times*, **89**, (30), 53–6.

Korniewicz, D.M., Kirwin, M., Cresci, K. *et al.* (1994) Barrier protection with examination gloves: double versus single. *American Journal of Infection Control,* **22,** 12–15.

Larson, E. (1988) A causal link between handwashing and risk of infection? Examination of the evidence. *Infection Control and Hospital Epidemiology,* **9,** 28–35.

Larson, E. (1995) APIC guidelines for handwashing and hand antisepsis in health care settings. *American Journal of Infection Control,* **23** (4), 251–69.

Leynadier, F., Pecquet, C. and Dry J. (1989) Anaphylaxis to latex during surgery. *Anaesthesia,* **44,** 547–5.

Lilly, H.A., Lowbury, E.J.L. and Wilkins, M.D. (1979) Limits to progressive reduction of resident skin bacteria by disinfection. *Journal of Clinical Pathology,* **32,** 382–5.

Lund, S., Jackson, J., Leggett, J. *et al.* (1994) Reality of glove use and handwashing in a community hospital. *American Journal of Infection Control,* **22** (6), 352–57.

Lynch, P., Jackson, M. and Nenner, V. (1992) *Monitoring and Preventing Blood Exposures for Health Care Workers,* Marvik Educational Services, San Diego.

Mackintosh, C.A. and Hoffman, P.N. (1984) An extended model for transfer of micro-organisms and the effect of alcohol disinfection. *Journal of Hygiene,* **92,** 345–55.

McLane, C., Chenelly, S., Sylwestrak, M.L. and Kirchoff, K.T. (1983) A nursing practice problem: failure to observe aseptic technique. *American Journal of Infection Control,* **11,** 178–82.

Mercier, C. (1994) Reducing the incidence of sharps injuries. *British Journal of Nursing,* **3** (17), 897–901.

Meers, P.D. and Leong, K.Y. (1989) Hot-air dryers. *Journal of Hospital Infection,* **14,** 169–71.

Morse, L.J. and Schonbeck, L.E. (1968) Hand lotions – a potential nosocomial hazard. *New England Journal of Medicine,* **278,** 376–78.

Olsen, R.J., Lynch, P., Coyle, M.B., *et al.* (1993) Examination gloves as barriers to hand contamination in clinical practice. *JAMA,* **270,** 350–53.

PHLS Hepatitis Subcommittee (1992) Exposure to hepatitis B virus: guidance on post-exposure prophylaxis, *CDR Review,* **2** (9), R97–R101.

Pottinger, J., Burns, S. and Manske, C. (1989) Bacterial carriage by artificial versus natural nails. *American Journal of Infection Control,* **17,** 340–40.

Redway, K., Knights, B., Bozoky, Z. and Theobald, A. (1994) Hand drying: a study of bacterial types associated with different hand drying methods and with hot air dryers.: University of Westminster: Association of Makers of Soft Tissue Papers. *Tech. Rep.*

Reybrouck, G. (1983) Role of the hands in the spread of nosocomial infections. *Journal of Hospital Infection,* **4,** 103–10.

Ridzon, R., Gallagher, K., Ciesielski, C., *et al.* (1997) Simultaneous transmission of human immunodeficiency virus and hepatitis C virus from a needlestick injury. *New England Journal of Medicine,* **336,** (13), 919–22.

Robinton, E.D. and Mood, E.W. (1968) A study of bacterial contaminants of cloth and paper towels. *American Journal of Public Health,* **58,** 1452–59.

Sanderson, P.J. and Weissler, S. (1992) Recovery of coliforms from the hands of nurses and patients; activities leading to contamination. *Journal of Hospital Infection*, **21**, 85–93.

Steere, A.C. and Mallison, G.F. (1975) Handwashing practices for the prevention of nosocomial infections. *Ann. Internal Medicine*, **83**, 683–90.

Taylor, L.J. (1978) An evaluation of handwashing techniques – 1. *Nursing Times*, **74**, 54–5.

Vickers, J., Painter, M.J., Heptonstall, J., Yusof, J.H.M. and Craske, J. (1994) Hepatitis B outbreak in a drug trials unit; investigation and recommendations. *CDR Review*, **4**, (1), R1–R4.

Wurtz, R., Moye, G. and Jovanovic, B. (1994) Handwashing machines, handwashing compliance, and potential for cross-contamination. *American Journal of Infection Control*, **22** (4), 228–30.

Cleaning, disinfection and sterilisation | 10

Most HCWs today are used to working in a clean environment and using equipment that has been correctly decontaminated. Much equipment which is regularly used for invasive procedures is single-use disposable. The general public also expects that sterile equipment will be used on them if they undergo an invasive procedure. However it was not always like this in the UK. Prior to the acceptance of antisepsis and asepsis at the beginning of the twentieth century, many patients acquired infections in hospital. In other parts of the world, where health care resources are limited, a lot of equipment, which in the West would be single-use disposable, is re-used (e.g. gloves, needles and syringes).

It is essential that HCWs have an understanding of the sterilisation, disinfection and cleaning of equipment in order that their practice is knowledge based. Generally, it is much more important to keep health care environments cleaner than people's own homes, as there is a far greater risk of cross-infection in health care environments, e.g. nursing and residential homes.

DECONTAMINATION

This is a general term which includes, sterilisation, disinfection and cleaning.

Definitions

Sterilisation

This is a process that is used to remove completely all micro-organisms, including bacterial spores.

Disinfection

This is a process that is used to reduce the number of micro-organisms, but not usually bacterial spores, to a level which is not harmful to health. There is either environmental or skin disinfection.

Antiseptic

An antiseptic is a non-toxic disinfectant used on skin and living tissue.

Cleaning

This is a process that physically removes contaminants including dust, soil and organic matter. Cleaning is usually a prerequisite to disinfection and sterilisation, as it removes organic matter which can protect organisms.

Decontamination methods

Micro-organisms can be transmitted to people from instruments, equipment or from the environment. For this reason health care premises must be clean and all instruments and equipment must be decontaminated between each use, and before they are sent for service or repair, even when there is no visible contamination. The level of decontamination is dependent on what the equipment is used for and the level of contamination.

Sterilisation

Sterilisation can be achieved by physical methods, such as heating in an autoclave (moist heat) or a hot air oven (dry heat), ionizing irradiation, or other methods involving steam and chemicals, e.g. ethylene oxide gas.

   The simplest of these methods and the one that is most readily accessible to HCWs is autoclaving. Autoclaves use steam under pressure: the atmospheric pressure is raised which means that instead of water boiling at 100°C (which it does at normal atmospheric pressure), water can be made to boil at much higher temperatures. The two temperatures commonly used in autoclaves are 121°C and 134°C. Steam at these higher temperatures destroys spores in 15 and 3 minutes, respectively. There are however a number of items, such as fibre-optic endoscopes and equipment made from some plastics, which are heat sensitive and cannot be processed in this way. For these items gaseous sterilisation with ethylene oxide is an option, but few health care centres, including large hospitals, have such a facility; cycles are long, and on the whole processing in this way is impractical. In these situations disinfectants are the only alternative.

At present, much of the sterile equipment used is single use disposable, e.g. needles and syringes. Other equipment, such as that used by most operating departments, is sent to central areas for sterilisation. However, this is not always the case in the community where many HCWs are now spending a lot of their time decontaminating equipment before sterilising them in bench top autoclaves. Sterilisers should conform to British Standard 3970. They should perform an automatic cycle and have a door lock to ensure that the cycle is complete before the equipment can be removed from the steriliser.

Re-using single use equipment
It is vitally important that equipment which is intended for single patient use is not re-sterilised and used on another patient (some areas have started to do this in the name of economy). If this is done HCWs must realise that the decontamination process may cost more in time and materials than the item itself. Decontamination may cause the item to malfunction and the manufacturer's liability is lost if the user takes on the responsibility of decontamination.

Disinfection

Disinfection is best achieved by moist heat such as boiling, which kills all organisms except some bacterial spores and 'slow viruses' even in the presence of organic matter. Other methods are pasteurization and steam at subatmospheric pressure.

The ideal disinfectant should be effective against a wide range of micro-organisms. It should be stable, safe to use (i.e. non-toxic and non-sensitizing) and should not damage the equipment being disinfected. It should also be affordable or cost effective. Unfortunately, no such wonder disinfectant exists to date. Therefore, it is important before choosing a disinfectant that expert advice is given which ensures that the disinfectant chosen meets the requirements considered to be the most important. In the hospital such advice should be sought from the hospital infection control committee. Representatives from the infection control committee should also be included in the hospital's supplies users group. This will mean that expert advice is given before the hospital purchases any new piece of equipment. It will also ensure that if decisions are taken to replace a certain item with another manufactured elsewhere, that there is infection contol input into the choice of the replacment, and that the infection control committee is aware of any such change.

In the community there is not always an obvious place to go for advice, though any infection control practitioner should be able to give the appropriate advice. Also, the department of health, manufacturers of equipment, professional societies and some reference centres all give advice.

In the United States there is an approved list of disinfectants, unfortunately this is not the case in the UK, where anyone can test and market a product. It is therefore incumbent on the purchaser of any equipment to ensure that they find out how equipment should be decontaminated prior to purchase.

Chemical disinfection

This is generally a complicated procedure as there are so many factors to take into account; the disinfectant used, its concentration and half-life, the organisms to be disinfected, the time it will take and the corrosive effects of the disinfectant. Also micro-organisms vary in their sensitivities. Generally, Gram-positive bacteria are sensitive, Gram-negative less sensitive, tubercle bacilli quite resistant and bacterial spores very resistant. Viruses too vary in their response to disinfectants. For this reason, ideally disinfectants should only be used for disinfecting clean surfaces as they often fail to penetrate organic matter, such as pus and faeces. They are also often inactivated by organic matter, some detergents, hard water and some materials, such as cork, rubber and plastic.

As disinfectants are chemicals, once activated they are often unstable and break down quite rapidly (Werry *et al.*, 1988). For this reason it is essential that fresh solutions are regularly made up, that disinfectants are never 'topped up' and that the container the new disinfectant is put in is itself clean. If disinfectants are not used diligently they may support the growth of certain micro-organisms and lead to gross contamination of instruments and equipment and the very real potential for cross-infection.

COSHH

It is the responsibility of employers to ensure that work practices, including methods of decontamination are safe to patient/clients and staff. Staff can also reduce the risk by ensuring that they follow safe practice guidelines. Pathogenic micro-organisms and many of the disinfectants used to destroy them are identified as hazardous substances under COSHH regulations (HSE, 1988). For this reason a COSHH assessment must be carried out on any procedure where a disinfectant will be used. This will include the substance to be used, the nature of its use, the likely exposure of people to the substance (staff and patients/clients) and measures to be taken to limit exposure.

The emphasis of the COSHH regulations is on preventing exposure to hazardous substances. This means that first, there should be an assessment to see whether the substance being evaluated does need to be used, or whether there is an alternative, such as using single use disposable items, or sending equipment elsewhere to be decontaminated by another system. If the substance does need to be used the employer must take steps to ensure that all safe working procedures and protective clothing are available, used and monitored. Protective clothing will generally need to be worn, often gloves, face/eye protection and a plastic apron. When necessary the exposure of employees should be monitored. The employer also has a duty to ensure that their employees and any other non-employees on the premises understand the safety issues.

As disinfectants are corrosive to equipment their use is often followed by a rinse. This leads to the potential for recontamination of the equipment. Some disinfectants act much quicker than others, for example chlorine granules take two minutes whereas glutaraldehyde may take several hours, depending on its use. It is crucial that the manufacturer's instructions are followed at all times to ensure disinfection is correctly achieved. Prior to disinfecting an item it is important that it is thoroughly cleaned; disinfectants do not penetrate organic matter, and if equipment is not cleaned it may not be adequately disinfected.

Do's and don'ts of disinfection

Do

Do follow the manufacturer's guidelines.
Do measure disinfectant and water correctly.
Do use a clean dry bucket/bowl.
Do wash dirt away first before using disinfectant.
Do throw away your disinfectant solution when the day's work is done.
Do remember that incorrectly stored disinfectants can become contaminated by bacteria and may actually spread infection.

Don't

Don't use disinfectant to sterilise.
Don't store cleaning tools in disinfectant.
Don't 'top up' disinfectant solutions.
Don't use yesterday's solutions, make up fresh.
Don't mix two disinfectants together.
Don't add detergent.
Don't expect disinfectant to make dirt safe.

Cleaning

Cleaning is an aspect of our lives that we take for granted. We wash ourselves, our clothes and generally expect the environment in which we live and work to be clean. In health care, general cleaning is all that is required on a daily basis. Thorough cleaning removes the majority of

micro-organisms present in the environment (Ayliffe *et al.*, 1993). In the hospital, general practitioner's surgery or health centre, general domestic cleaning of floors, walls and other surfaces such as furniture and shelves is all that is required. Detergent is generally adequate. Additional disinfectants are only necessary if surfaces have been contaminated with material such as blood, pus or faeces in which case the area should be cleaned as for spillages (Chapter 9).

It is important to realize that any equipment that is used for cleaning, such as mops, brushes and cloths must also be cleaned and dried after use.

Good cleaning practice

Good cleaning practice includes a number of activities.

- Use a clean, dry container.
- Use correctly diluted cleaning solution.
- Use clean and dry mops or cloths. Wear appropriate protective clothing.
- Avoid the use of excess fluid to clean as this prevents proper drying of surfaces.
- Change cleaning solution at regular intervals to avoid recontamination of surfaces with soiled fluid.
- Cleaning solutions must penetrate any soiled area for effective cleaning.
- Pour away used solution carefully into sluice hopper or designated utility area and avoid splashing.
- The cleaned area must be dried either physically by using disposable paper towels or naturally via good ventilation.
- After cleaning, hands should be washed and dried.

Risk categories and effective decontamination

How and with what an item should be decontaminated is dependent on a number of factors. In order to simplify the procedure items can be classified as below.

High risk items

Items in close contact with a break in the skin or mucous membrane or one that is introduced into a sterile body cavity, such as surgical instruments, intrauterine devices and stitch cutters, require **sterilisation**.

Medium risk items

Items in contact with intact mucous membranes or non-intact skin, such as endoscopes, require **sterilisation/disinfection**

Low risk items

Items in contact with intact skin or that do not come into close contact with the patient, such as BP cuffs, ear syringe nozzles and mattresses require **cleaning and drying.**

All other items that are not in close contact with the patient/client, such as sinks, walls and floors present a minimal risk and only require cleaning.

Sterilising items

Many items used by HCWs are single use disposable. However some items, notably surgical instruments are reusable once sterilised. Moist heat is the best method of sterilising such used equipment in the health care setting. Most provider units have access to central sterile supply departments (CSSD), where large autoclaves operate and sterilise wrapped instruments.

If HCWs have access to CSSDs they should use them, as they generally provide an efficient quick service and are run and monitored by staff who understand how and why equipment needs to be sterilised. They cut down on the time HCWs take on decontaminating equipment, as most CSSDs treat all equipment as potentially infectious, and all equipment that enters the department is put through a tunnel washer which heat-disinfects the equipment so that it is safe for staff to handle and wrap prior to sterilisation.

In some areas staff do not have ready access to CSSDs and they need to sterilize their own equipment. Various sterilisers that autoclave equipment, are available on the market. The most important aspect to remember is that to date there are no bench top autoclaves which sterilise wrapped instruments. All equipment which goes into these autoclaves (Little Sisters, Matrons) must go in unwrapped so that the steam can penetrate and effectively sterilise the equipment. It is best to use an autoclave with an automatic cycle and temperature and pressure indicators.

Before sterilisation, all equipment must be cleaned thoroughly to remove all visible deposits. This is best achieved if the equipment is scrubbed with hot water and detergent. The HCW performing this task must ensure they have on the correct protective clothing which, in most cases will be thick household style gloves (Marigold), a plastic apron and, if using a scrubbing brush or if there is any risk of splashing to the face or eyes, face or eye protection. The equipment should then be placed in the autoclave in such a way as to ensure that all the surfaces will be exposed to steam. There are different time temperature combinations to use to ensure sterilisation (Table 10.1), and the highest temperature compatible with the equipment to be sterilised should be used.

Table 10.1 Temperature combinations to ensure sterilisation

Temperature (°C)	Minimum hold time in minutes
134–138	3 mins[a]
126–129	10 mins[a]
121–124	15 mins[a]
160–180	20–120[b]

[a] moist heat
[b] dry heat

Ideally, the brushes used to clean the equipment should be autoclaved with the equipment. If this is not possible (if the plastic cannot be autoclaved), they can be washed and disinfected and stored dry after use.

Consideration of appropriate methods of decontamination should always be given to any equipment that is being bought. There is nothing worse than using a piece of equipment only to realize that you do not have access to an effective, quick and cheap method of decontamination.

It is essential that the autoclave is regularly serviced, and a service record is shown in Table 10.2.

Table 10.2 Service record for autoclave

Type of autoclave: ....
Make: .... Number: ....
Model: ....
Frequency of checks: ....
The autoclave maintenance company is: ....
Telephone: ....
Contact name: ....
Date for contract renewal: ....
The record of daily checks is kept by: ....

Check list for using sterilised equipment

Before treatment
- Ensure that all relevant equipment has been sterilised.
- Disinfect surfaces and place clean coverings over equipment to prevent contamination.

During treatment
- Follow UICP:
  - wash hands;

- treat all patients as potentially infectious;
- perform a risk assessment and wear the appropriate protective clothing;
- handle sharps safely.

After treatment
- clean instruments thoroughly;
- sterilize all instruments;
- dispose of sharps and other waste safely;
- clean work surfaces.

Chemical disinfection of instruments

The use of chemical disinfectants is to be discouraged, principally because it is very difficult to check their effectiveness. Process times can be many hours, and there must be adherence to COSHH regulations. However, there are still some instances when the only method of decontamination is by chemical disinfection.

Checklist for using chemical disinfectants

Before treatment
- Ensure that you are only using equipment that has been chemical disinfected to ensure that all relevant equipment has been correctly disinfected prior to use.
- Disinfect surfaces and place clean coverings over equipment to prevent contamination.

During treatment
- follow UICPs:
  - wash hands;
  - treat all patients as potentially infectious;
  - perform a risk assessment and wear the appropriate protective clothing;
  - handle sharps safely.

After treatment
- clean instruments thoroughly;
- ensure that disinfection is necessary and that you are using the correct disinfectant, and that it is fresh;
- check the COSHH assessment;
- wear the correct protective clothing;
- immerse equipment for the correct length of time, use a timer;

- rinse equipment after use, ensure that you are not recontaminating the equipment;
- dispose of sharps and other waste safely;
- clean work surfaces.

Different chemical disinfectants

Alcohol

There are different types of alcohol used for chemical disinfection such as 70% isopropyl alcohol, 70% industrial methylated spirits, alcohol impregnated wipes (e.g. Sterets and Alcowipes). Alcohol is effective against bacteria (including the tubercle bacilli) and fungi but not bacterial spores. Ethanol (IMS at concentrations of 90%) is effective against most categories of virus. However isopropanol is not effective. Alcohol has a rapid action, but it is flammable and does not penetrate organic matter well. Therefore, cleaning is essential first. It is most useful as a skin disinfectant as it dries rapidly, but care must be taken with diathermy or electrical equipment.

Chlorhexidine

Chlorhexidine is produced under various brand names such as Hibiscrub, Hibitane and Savlon. It has a good fungicidal activity and is active against Gram-positive organisms. It is less effective against Gram-negative organisms, and is not active against the tubercle bacilli or bacterial spores. It has limited activity against viruses. Chlorhexidine is easily inactivated by organic matter, and is most useful as a skin or mucous membrane disinfectant, but it should not come into contact with the brain, meninges or middle ear.

Detergent

Fairy liquid is an example of a detergent. It breaks up grease and dirt, and thereby makes it easier for disinfectants to work.

Glutaraldehyde

Examples of glutaraldehyde include: Cidex, Guigasept and Asep. It has good bactericidal, virucidal and fungicidal activity, and is active against tubercle bacilli in 60 minutes. It is also active against bacterial spores, but it is slow (10 hours). There is little inactivation by organic matter, but it penetrates slowly. It is highly irritant to skin and mucosa, (Ayliffe, Coate and Hoffman, 1993). It is currently used by many areas to disinfect equipment that is heat labile, as it is relatively cheap. However, it is toxic and requires different immersion times, dependent on the perceived infection risk to patients, therefore cross-contamination has occurred.

Hydrogen peroxide
Hydrogen peroxide has a wide range of bactericidal, virucidal and fungicidal activity, but its activity is greatly reduced by organic matter, and is poor against bacterial spores and tubercle bacilli. It has low toxicity and irritancy but it is corrosive to some metals. It is used for ophthalmic equipment.

Hypochlorites
Examples of hypochlorites include: Milton, Domestos and Presept. They have a wide range of bactericidal, virucidal, sporicidal and fungicidal activity. There is rapid action, but care should be taken not to mix strong acids with them as chlorine gas will be released. Therefore they should not be used on urine. This is the disinfectant of choice for viruses, as it has a rapid action and is cheap.

Paracetic acid
Nu-cidex and Steris are types of paracetic acid which have a wide range of bactericidal, virucidal, sporicidal and fungicidal activity. They are also effective against tubercle bacilli, have a rapid action and low irritancy. In some areas they are used in preference to glutaraldehyde as they guarantee sterility, at certain times, much quicker than glutaraldehyde. Paracetic Acid has a short life once activated and it is expensive. The effect of paracetic acid on equipment is still uncertain (Babb and Bradley, 1995).

Phenolics
Hycolin and Clearsol are phenolics which have a wide range of bactericidal activity including tubercle bacilli. However, there is poor activity against bacterial spores. They are irritant to the skin, absorbed by rubber and plastics and should not therefore be used to disinfect equipment that is used on skin or mucous membranes.

Service and repair

Any equipment that has been in contact with patients/clients or used for invasive procedures, when it may come into contact with blood or body fluids, is a potential source of infection to any staff who may service or repair it. To comply with the Health and Safety at Work Act, 1974, all such equipment must be decontaminated before it is inspected or repaired. 1993 guidance (NHS Management Executive, 1993) states that a certificate demonstrating the method of decontamination should always accompany any item requiring servicing or repair (Figure 10.1).

Table 10.3 A–Z of equipment decontamination

Equipment	Method	Comments/Instructions
Airways	Disposable	Discard as clinical waste after use
Ambu-bags	Use a filter	Change after each patient
	Sterilise	Autoclave
Ampoules	Not necessary	
Anaesthetic masks	Disposable	Discard as clinical waste
	Sterilise	Autoclave
Auriscopes	Clean	After each use
	Disinfect	70% Alcohol wipe
Baby bottles	Disposable	After each use
	Disinfect	125 ppm available chlorine for one hour or boil for five mins
Baby changing mats	Disposable paper towel	Change after each use
	Clean	After each use with detergent. If visibly soiled treat as spillages. If covering no longer intact discard
Baby scales	Disposable paper towel	Change after each use
	Clean	After each use
Baths	Clean	After each use
Bath hoists	Clean	After each use
Bedframes	Clean	After each use
Bedpans/potties		
● hospital	Washer/disinfector	After each use 80°C for 1 min
	Disposable	Macerator
		Clean carriers
● home	Clean	Contents into toilet
	Disposable	Contents into toilet, then into clinical waste.
Bowls		
● surgical	Sterilise	Autoclave
● washing	Clean	After each use, store inverted
Cervical caps	Sterilise (steam)	After each use
Clinical thermometers	Use disposable sheath	After each use
	Clean	After each use
	Disinfect	After each client use alcohol-impregnated wipe.
Commodes	Clean	After each use
	Clean/disinfect	If visibly soiled
Crockery/cutlery	Disinfect	After each use in dish washer or hot water and detergent
Diaphragms and practice caps	Sterilise	After each use
Dressing Trolleys	Clean	At beginning of day or if visibly soiled
Duvets		
● PVC Covered	Clean	After each client
● fabric	Wash	After each client
● cover	Wash	After each client and when soiled
Endoscopes	See above	
Examination couches	Disposable paper towel	Dispose after each use
	Clean	End of each session If cover no longer intact discard
Floors, furniture		
● wet	Clean	
● dry	Vacuum or use dust attracting mops	

Table 10.3 A–Z of equipment decontamination

Equipment	Method	Comments/Instructions
Flower vases	Clean	
Hands	UICP (Chapter 9)	
Incubators	Clean	After each baby
Instruments	Sterilise	
Jugs		
• hospital	Sterilise	Autoclave
	Washer/disinfector	After each use
• home	Clean	
Laryngoscope		
• handles	Clean	After each use
• blade	Sterilise	After each use
Mannequins	Disinfect	Between each use with alcohol impregnated wipe
Mattresses	Clean	After each patient and when soiled[b]
Mops	Wash	Daily
Nailbrushes	Sterilise	After each use
Nebulizers	Clean	After each use
	Disposable	After each patient
Ophthalmic prisms	Disinfect	After each use
Pillows	Clean	After each use: if cover no longer intact, discard
Razors		
• electric	Clean/disinfect	Not recommended for communal use in hospital/residential homes
• disposable	Dispose as sharps	After each use
Scissors	Disinfect/sterilise	After each use
Spatula	Single use disposable	
Specula		
• vaginal	Disposable	After each use
	Sterilise	After each use
Spirometer	Change mouthpiece	After each client
Spoons	Single use disposable	
Stethoscopes	Disinfect	After each use
Suction		
• bottles	Use disposable liners	
	Sterilise	After each use
• tubing	Disposable	
• filter	Disposable	Three monthly or when discoloured
Toys		
• hard	Clean	
• soft	Wash	
Urinals	Washer/disinfector	After each use
	Disposable	

Any equipment which is contaminated with blood or body fluids must be treated as for spillages, see Chapter 9.

*Mattresses: to check if in a good state of repair there should be i) no visible staining and ii) they should be impermeable to fluids. To test, open the mattress and check filling is dry to the touch. If it is, place a paper towel beneath the cover press down for ten seconds, pour 30 mls of water onto the area and press for a further 30 seconds and examine the paper towel for moisture.

Equipment decontamination

A summary of equipment decontamination is given in Table 10.3.
An example decontamination certificate is shown below:

Declaration of contamination status

Make and description of equipment/item:..

Model/serial/batch no:...

A[a]   This equipment/item could not be decontaminated. The nature of risk
       and safety precautions to be adopted are:

       ....

       ....

B[a]   This equipment/item has been cleaned and decontaminated.
       The method of decontamination was:

       ....

       ....

C[a]   This equipment/item has not been used in an invasive procedure or been in
       contact with blood, other body fluids, or pathological samples.
       It has been cleaned in preparation for inspection, servicing or repair.

D[a]   Has the equipment been suitably prepared to ensure
       safe handling/transport?   YES/NO
       I declare that I have taken all reasonable steps to ensure the
       accuracy of the above information.
       Authorized signature:...Date:...
       Position held:...From:..

       [a]Please delete as appropriate

Figure 10.1 Inspection, servicing or repair of all equipment

REFERENCES

Ayliffe, G.A.J., Coates, D. and Hoffman, P.N. (1993) *Chemical Disinfection in Hospital*, PHLS, London.

Babb, J. and Bradley, C.R. (1995) A review of glutaraldehyde alternative. *British Journal of Theatre Nursing*, **5**, (7).

Health & Safety Executive (HSE) (1988) *Control of Substances Hazardous to Health Regulations*, HMSO, London.

NHS Management Executive (1993) *Decontamination of Equipment Prior to Inspection, Service or Repair*, HSG(93)26 HMSO, London.

Werry, C., Lawrence, J.M. and Sanderson, P.J. (1988) Contamination of detergent cleaning solutions during hospital cleaning. *Journal of Hospital Infection*, **11**, 44–9.

FURTHER READING

Department of Health (NHS Procurement Directorate) (1990) A Further Evaluation of Portable Steam Sterilizers for Unwrapped Instruments and Utensils. Health Equipment Information, No.196. *Tech. Rep.*

Health & Safety Executive (HSE) (1992) *Occupational Exposure Standards: Guidance Note*, EH40/92, HMSO, London.

NHS Procurement Directorate (1996) *A Further Evaluation of Transportable Steam Sterilizers for Unwrapped Instruments and Utensils. Health Equipment Information 196*, HMSO, London.

UK Health Departments (1994) *Dry heat sterilizers: purchase, maintenance and use*, SAB(94)23, HMSO, London.

11

Waste disposal

The western world is a society of consumers, who are constantly demanding more new produce, thus creating waste. Although the twentieth century has seen huge technological advances in waste disposal, and there have been undoubted improvements, there remains a problem about what to do with all the waste produced through technology and modern living. Over the past decade many people have become increasingly concerned about the amount of waste human beings are producing and what the world is going to do with it.

NHS WASTE

The NHS itself creates many millions of tonnes of waste a year. This waste is seen by the general public as offensive and aesthetically unacceptable, therefore they regard the improper management of clinical waste as environmentally and visibly objectionable (Griffiths, 1989). Consequently, incidents during the collection and disposal of waste lead both operatives and the general population to express concern.

It is, however, accepted by many that operatives and the general public do not realise that it is necessary for intact skin to be pierced or injured and for micro-organisms present in the waste to come into contact with the damaged skin, conjunctiva or mucosa in sufficient numbers before any cross-infection can occur. The organisms also need to be of sufficient virulence to cause disease even when they have gained a portal of entry. The immune status and susceptibility of the individual also needs to be considered.

The actual dangers of contracting an infection from clinical (yellow bag) waste is believed to be small by many microbiologists (Carlisle, 1989; Ayliffe, 1994). Therefore it is important not to overstate any hazards. Used dressings, incontinence pads, sputum containers, urine and stoma bags could potentially present a risk of infection, especially if contaminated with blood. However, organisms recovered from these items such as

Pseudomonas aeruginosa, *Proteus* spp., *Staphylococcus aureus*, *Strepto-coccus faecalis* and coliforms are found in the normal human body flora and the environment (Gibbs, 1991). They all have the potential to cause infection in certain individuals, but not in all circumstances. The above wastes, especially large amounts, must be disposed of in an acceptable manner and because of the aesthetic considerations, disposal via house-hold rubbish as a routine is no longer considered acceptable.

Waste disposal operatives frequently report injuries caused by sharps concealed in domestic wastes, and a real hazard is cross-infection following a sharps injury with a needle contaminated with blood. Blood borne viruses, such as HIV and the hepatitis viruses, can be transmitted by a contaminated sharp. It has been estimated that although it requires at least 0.10 ml of infected blood to transmit HIV, only 0.00004 ml of blood is required to transmit hepatitis B, but the virus can survive in the dried state (BMA, 1990). Landfill sites are also not vandal proof, so there is a potential risk to the public if such waste ends up on a landfill site (Carlisle, 1989). The increased usage of single use disposable items in health care has emphasised the problems of waste disposal plus the associated risks (real and perceived), and the costs.

The cost of disposal is enormous, and steps will have to be taken to control the amount of waste being produced. This is not only because of the associated costs but because there is a needless consumption of raw materials and products. Much of the waste could be recycled, but segrega-tion and recycling are still not considered as normal practice in the UK health setting (Muir Gray, 1994; Ayliffe, 1994). Correct segregation of waste could save trusts many thousands of pounds a year (Mercier and Ellam, 1996).

To achieve any lasting change in how waste is managed, the discussion needs to be at national, health authority and trust management level. A major shift in the way waste is managed could reduce costs, minimise waste produced and maximise recycling techniques. It has been reported in Germany (Daschner, 1993) that, by discussing the re-use of single use items, recycling materials, using incineration to produce cost effective energy, using biodegradable products and encouraging manufacturers to produce re-usable products, savings can be made.

A European Union (EU) packaging directive has had further impact on the costs of waste management in the the UK in the form of a levy on producers to fund the monitoring of the use of raw materials in packaging and their subsequent recycling. The target is to recover and recycle between 45 and 65% of all packaging from all sources by the year 2000 (Howarth, 1994).

Recovering is defined as re-use, recycling and incineration with energy recovery. It is accepted that a scheme such as this will be expensive for the health care industry and health packaging. However, a group has been set up to look at minimising the amount of packaging for health care products and to encourage recovery of packaging (Howarth, 1994).

THE LEGISLATIVE FRAMEWORK

At a national level, responsibility for laying down the standards for waste disposal and recycling lies with the Department of the Environment. At a local level, until April 1 1996, the Waste Disposal Authority (WDA) or Waste Regulatory Authority (WRA) and the Collection Authority implemented a waste disposal policy. In England the relevant WRA was the county council, whilst in Wales, Northern Ireland and Scotland it was the district council. The collection authorities who are responsible for collection of household refuse are always the district councils.

A new Environment Agency for England and Wales has been in existence since April 1 1996. It has been created to provide a more comprehensive approach to management of the environment by combining the regulation of land, air and water. It brings together the National Rivers Authority, Her Majesty's Inspectorate of Pollution and the WRA. This has made the WRA independent of local councils.

The important regulatory and statutory functions of the WRA are stated in the Control of Pollution (Amendment) Act, 1989 (HMSO, 1989) and this role is further supported by other supporting legislation, the most important of which is the Environment Protection Act 1990 (HMSO, 1990). The Commission of the European Community (EC) considers waste control, recovery and safe disposal as central to its environmental protection strategy. Their directives are implemented in the UK through the Environmental Protection Act 1990 and The Control of Pollution (Amendment) Act 1989.

The Environment Protection Act, 1990 (Section 75; sub-section 2–4) defines waste.

- 'Waste' includes:
  - any substance which constitutes a scrap metal or an effluent or unwanted surplus substance arising from the application of any process;
  - any substance or article which requires to be disposed of as being broken, worn out, contaminated or otherwise spoiled, but it does not include a substance which is an explosive within the meaning of the Explosives Act, 1875.
- Anything which is discarded or otherwise dealt with as if it were waste shall be presumed to be waste unless the contrary is proved.
- 'Controlled waste' means household, industrial and commercial waste or any such waste.

The Environment Protection Act, 1990, gives a broad definition of 'household, industrial and commercial waste' and the Controlled Waste Regulations, 1992, (HMSO, 1992) describe these categories in more detail within a series of schedules. Schedule 2 of the Control Waste Regulations, 1992, sets out the types of household waste for which a charge for collection may be made. This includes yellow bag waste for incineration from a property, caravan or vessel used as living accommodation. Charges are at the discretion of district councils and are usually waived if householders are in receipt of state benefit.

Since September 1 1996 a new definition of 'special wastes' has been in existence including certain wastes from human health care and/or related research. All special wastes are given a six digit code.

Clinical waste produced by householders on domestic premises is exempt from the Waste Management: Duty of Care 1991, regulations (HMSO, 1991). This may lead to confusion in the community where patients are being nursed at home or providing self care, e.g. diabetics, and will be considered in more detail below.

Categories of clinical waste

Category A

This category includes all human tissue, including blood (whether infected or not), animal carcasses and tissue from veterinary centres, hospitals or laboratories, and all related swabs and dressings. It also includes waste materials, where the assessment indicates a risk to staff handling them, for example from infectious disease cases. Soiled surgical dressings, swabs and all other soiled waste from treatment areas are included in category A as well.

Category B

Discarded syringes, needles, cartridges, broken glass and other sharp instruments are in category B.

Category C

This category includes microbiological cultures and potentially infected waste from pathology departments (laboratory and post-mortem rooms) and other clinical or research laboratories.

Category D

Certain pharmaceutical and chemical wastes are included in category D.

Category E

This category includes items used to dispose of urine, faeces and other bodily secretions, and excretions assessed as not falling within the first section. This includes used disposable bedpan liners, incontinence pads, stoma bags and urine containers.

The Duty of Care (HMSO, 1991)

The Environment Protection Act (section 34), 1990, imposes a *'Duty of Care'* on all those responsible for producing waste, and imposes criminal liability on individuals responsible for producing waste. The 'duty of care' is an approved code of practice and can therefore be submitted as evidence of good practice in court. Compliance with the 'duty of care' means that all waste can be tracked back to source.

Clinical waste regulations

These regulations state that:

- a disposal contract must be arranged with an authorized carrier;
- a written description of the waste should be prepared (4 copies) – this is the consignment note;
- the relevant copies of the consignment note will travel with the waste;
- the relevant copies will be given to the consignee on delivery;
- one copy will be returned to the agency who has the waste contract;
- the waste will be disposed of on an authorised site;
- copies of the consignment notes are kept for two years.

Section 33 of the Environment Protection Act, 1990, applies to treating, keeping and disposing of controlled waste stating in Section 33(1c) that a person shall not: 'treat, keep or dispose of controlled waste in a manner likely to cause pollution of the environment of harm to human health'. Registration of waste carriers is controlled by the Control of Pollution Amendment Act, 1989 (HMSO, 1989).

Annex B of the 'duty of care' determines who are the waste producers. An item may become waste either by being changed in some way such as during delivery of care or by a decision of the holder that something is no longer required. If an action is required the waste producer will be the person committing the action and must accept responsibility for the safe disposal of the waste, e.g. used needles and syringes must be placed directly into a sharps container approved by UN 3291. Where clinical waste is generated in the community, usually the health care professional creating the waste is easily identified and they ensure the correct disposal of the waste via registered waste disposal services (usually the district council). The issue becomes blurred when people are involved in self care. Although the waste generated may be classed as clinical waste, and subject to the 'duty of care', individual householders are exempt and can dispose of the waste in normal household rubbish; the disposal of needles and syringes in this way being of particular concern.

The household is undeniably the producer of the waste, but it could be argued that the person who prescribes the particular mode of self care has a responsibility under the 'duty of care' to ensure waste products of this care or treatment are disposed of safely. This should take the form of patient information, education and provision of the physical means for correct and safe disposal. The legal framework is complex, but there is a summary in Table 11.1.

Table 11.1 Summary of the legal framework

The Environment Protection Act (1990)
Section 34 includes a duty of care in relation to waste management.
Section 75 sub-section 2–4 defines waste.
Waste Management: A Duty of Care (1991)
An approved code of practice.
Compliance with this code of practice would be viewed in a court of law as evidence of good practice in waste management.
Controlled Waste Regulations (1992)
Collection authorities are given leave to charge for collection.
The Special Waste Regulations (1996)
This defines special waste, and is more stringent about consignment notes.

Health and safety legislation and special waste

The Health and Safety at Work Act 1974 (HMSO, 1974) applies to all work activities and requires employers to ensure as far as is reasonably practicable the health and safety of their employees and any other people who may be affected by the work activity. It also places the onus on employees to ensure safe working practices and to take advantage of the facilities provided for personal protection. To achieve this objective section 2(3) of the Act calls for written development of a health and safety policy. Included in this should be a policy for the safe disposal and handling of clinical waste. The framework for such a policy is set out in The Safe Disposal of Clinical Waste (Health and Safety Commission, 1992) and includes the following:

- identification of categories of waste;
- means of segregation;
- specification of containers used;
- storage;
- transport;
- training needs;
- personal protection;
- accident and incident reporting and follow-up;
- handling before disposal;
- spillages;
- final disposal of waste.

Complementary to this Act are the Control of Substances Hazardous to Health Regulations (Health and Safety Commission, 1994). These regulations specifically require that risk assessments are made for all hazardous substances likely to be encountered as a result of a work activity.

The Management of Health and Safety at Work, Regulations, 1992, require the employer to carry out risk assessments of all work activities (HMSO, 1974). In the case of waste disposal, risk assessment should already be carried out as a requirement under the COSHH regulations. These include: Control of Substances Hazardous to Health Regulations, 1994; general COSHH approved code of practice; *and* biological agents approved code of practice (Health and Safety Commission, 1994). Finally, details about reporting of injuries, diseases and dangerous occurrences are contained in the Reporting of Injuries, Diseases and Dangerous Occurrence Regulations, 1985 (HMSO, 1985).

The categories of special waste form the foundation of local risk assessment. At local level, a list of places where waste arises is useful and allows for more meaningful risk assessment when considering how to handle the waste, how to deal with accidental spillage (Figure 11.1), or any injuries sustained. An overall waste policy should reflect local circumstances, the COSHH assessments being an integral part of its development.

Where nursing care is taking place in the home the Royal College of Nursing suggests in their leaflet entitled *Disposal of Health Care Waste in the Community* (RCN, 1994) that the person responsible for the nursing care plan must include an assessment for the disposal of waste and record this in writing.

Meaningful risk assessment requires assessment of the perceived risk compared to the actual risk and will comprise information from patient's case notes, other professional colleagues involved in the care, microbiological advice and reference to local waste policies. Knowledge of the site where the waste arises (e.g. hospital, ward, home, GP surgery, dental surgery, clinic, tattooist, veterinary surgery or funeral parlour) will give

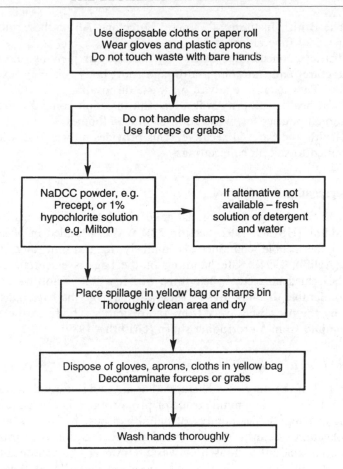

Figure 11.1 Spillage of clinical waste

an indication of the categories of waste for disposal and possible additional risk factors.

Additional guidelines are available for the producers of clinical waste and may be obtained from the following groups:

- The British Veterinary Association which will give advice on the veterinary surgeon's duty of care in handling and dispensing of clinical waste.
- The British Dental Association which will advise on the control of cross-infection in dentistry and the health and safety law for dental practitioners.
- The Co-operative Funeral Service Managers' Association; The British Institute of Embalmers; The National Association of Funeral Directors

and The British Institute of Funeral Directors. All of these will advise on aspects of funeral service.

- The district councils issue bylaws to regulate ear piercing, electrolysis, acupuncture and tattooing, although not body piercing except in London. They also issue advice on waste disposal.
- The local health authority will advise on infection control policies and operational policies for registration of nursing homes.
- The Health and Safety Executive. This provides information which can be adapted to suit all care settings.

Waste segregation and disposal

Prior to disposal, segregation must take place, and this is achieved via colour coding (HMSO, 1992, Section 22). Waste, if sealed in plastic bags or any impermeable container, is unlikely to transmit any infection present (Ayliffe, 1994). Safe handling of the bags is essential, and they should be sealed correctly when three quarters full. Knotting or taping bags is preferable to using tags as these can damage the bag. Bags should be held by the neck well away from the operative's body to prevent any possible injury from a protruding sharp (Griffiths, 1989).

Disposal of waste in the community

Sections 1–7 of the duty of care states that anything unusual in waste can pose a problem, as can anything out of proportion. This is relevant when disposing of nappies. The number of nappies disposed of into a household waste collection system in the average domestic situation is in proportion to the normal amount of household waste. However in a child health clinic for example, this number is out of proportion and should therefore be classed as clinical waste, to be incinerated, and placed in yellow bags.

Guidelines, agreed between WRAs and ICPs, state that if the amount of yellow bag (for incineration) waste generated is more than a quarter of a full size yellow bag a week, this should be disposed of by arranging a collection service by the local council. If less than a quarter of a full size yellow bag a week, the waste should be placed in a plastic bag, sealed, and then disposed of in the normal way as household waste.

Waste segregation by the colour coding system

Black bags
These are used for waste paper, packaging and some food waste. Exceptions include confidential papers, e.g. patient information, and it is good practice for each bag to be labelled with the area of origin, dated and sealed before final disposal in landfill sites.

Clear plastic bags or special boxes
These are used for aerosols, glassware and cans. Each bag/box should be labelled as above. This waste must be stored in a locked area to prevent access by unauthorised personnel and possible tampering. Final disposal is to a landfill site.

Yellow bags
These are used for:

- clinical waste as previously defined, dressings, swabs, used blood bags and amputated limbs;
- disposables when the patient has a known infection;
- confidential papers.

The yellow bags must comply to performance specifications set out by the NHS Supplies Authority (HSC, 1992), and they must be a minimum of 225 gauge. Heavy duty bags (800 gauge) are available for disposal of large items such as limbs, alternatively, such items may be double bagged. Also, all bags must fit the holding receptacle properly.

This waste must be stored in a locked area, which should be constructed of impervious materials to facilitate cleaning should there be any spillages. The waste should be collected as soon as possible to prevent any further risk of tampering or infestation by rodents or insects. Also, it is recommended that when waste is stored in bulk for up to one week, refrigerated storage may be needed (HSC, 1992).

Yellow sharps containers
These should conform to UN 3291 (formerly British Standard 7320) and should be used for all sharps including broken glass (BSI 1990). Exceptions to this are sharps in contact with the administration of cytotoxic drugs or radioactive substances.

Sharps containers must be locked and correctly sealed when three quarters full so that the contents cannot escape. They must not be placed in yellow bags for disposal, as incorrectly closed containers may allow sharps to escape, which may penetrate the bag and injure the disposal worker. Sharps containers should be stored and collected as for yellow bags. Further information on sharps is given in Chapter 9.

Cytotoxic, pharmaceutical and radioactive wastes
Methods of disposal of these wastes will vary according to local policy. The onus is on the HCWs to familiarise themselves with the disposal services available in their area. Final disposal of the waste is to incineration.

Laboratory waste

This is autoclaved prior to disposal to make it safe.

Future disposal of waste

The problems associated with the disposal of waste, particularly health care waste, will remain, mainly because of the public perception of risk and aesthetic considerations.

Suitable sites for landfill are decreasing and toxins can be produced from other processes such as incineration (Ayliffe, 1994).

In the future the waste disposal process will rely more and more on individual patient risk assessment. The safe and correct disposal of waste can only happen with the co-operation of all concerned, including health care workers, and a commitment by management to provide policy guidance, education and the correct equipment. More and more people are beginning to recycle waste in their own homes, and we need to begin to consider this as a viable option for the health service. We cannot continue to throw away plastics and other items. In the next few years we need to start seriously managing our waste.

FOOD HYGIENE IN HEALTH CARE

Everyone needs food and water to survive. We all undertake some form of food hygiene each day, by washing our hands before making food, placing food in refrigerators and cooking food. There are some basic rules for all food handlers to follow; this includes people who make a cup of tea or snack for a patient to world renowned chefs.

Basic food handling guidelines

Food handlers – personal hygiene

There are some basic rules for food handlers.

- Prior to undertaking any food handling, including the preparation of toast, sandwiches etc., hands must be washed thoroughly and dried. Hands must always be washed between handling different foods, e.g. between touching fresh meat and preparing vegetables.
- Any cuts or abrasions must be covered with a coloured waterproof plaster, and fingernails should be kept short and clean.
- Fingers should not be licked, and the food handler should avoid touching his hair or face when handling food.
- Avoid sneezing or coughing over food.
- Clean protective clothing should be worn.

- Any food handler suffering from sickness and/or diarrhoea, infected cuts or sores or infections of the eyes or ears must stop handling food and report to their manager. They should seek advice from their general practitioner or their occupational health department.
- Any food handlers who have been on holiday and have experienced diarrhoea or vomiting should report to their GP or the occupational health department prior to recommencing work.

Equipment and the environment

To ensure good food hygiene, it is essential that the equipment and environment are clean.

- All equipment that comes into contact with food products must be kept clean and in good condition.
- Areas where food is being prepared must have a washhand basin, soap and paper hand towels. Bins must be available for the disposal of paper towels. Washhand basins should not be used for washing food or cleaning equipment.
- Walls, floors, doors, windows, ceilings, woodwork and all other structures where food is prepared must be kept clean and in a good state of repair.
- Different cleaning cloths must be used for crockery, sinks, floors, etc.
- Waste must be disposed of safely in accordance with current legislation.
- Refrigerator temperatures should not exceed 8°C.
- Freezer temperatures should not exceed minus 18°C.
- Surfaces and cutlery should be cleaned thoroughly between preparing cooked and raw food. When possible, separate chopping boards should be used which are clearly labelled or colour coded, e.g. red for raw meat, blue for fish. When separate chopping boards are not available, utensils must be washed and dried thoroughly before cutting different types of food products.
- Tea towels must be kept clean, and should be washed at 60°C minimum.
- The use of dishwashers where possible is advisable. If they are not used, crockery and cutlery must be washed with hot soapy water, washing up gloves should be worn to enable the person who is washing up to use water as hot as possible.
- A regular cleaning schedule should be in place for ovens, hobs, microwaves, etc.
- Any infestation of rodents or insects should be dealt with promptly.

Food storage

There are various rules about food storage.

- Cooked food and diary products should be kept at the top of the refrigerator, above uncooked and raw food. Raw meats should not touch or drip onto other foods, e.g. salads. Meat should be kept separate from other food.

- Cooked and uncooked food should be kept separate.
- Food should be covered with cling film or kept in an airtight container.
- When freezing or chilling food, cooked food should be placed in the freezer within 90 minutes of cooking. In commercial premises a blast chiller is used to achieve this. Where large portions of food need to be chilled, it is wise to divide the food into smaller portions, thus enabling chilling to occur.
- Food must be covered and placed in a cool place before refrigerating or freezing and hot food should not be placed immediately into a refrigerator as it will raise the temperature of the refrigerator.
- Food should be labelled.

Cooking food

When cooking food, it is important to observe the following rules.

- When cooking meat, it should be checked to ensure that it is thoroughly cooked by skewering it to see if the juices run clear.
- When cooking stews or casseroles, ensure that the stew reaches boiling temperature and then simmers for 20 minutes.
- Any food that is reheated must be reheated thoroughly to ensure that it is piping hot throughout and the reheating of food should be avoided where ever possible.
- Frozen food must always be defrosted thoroughly prior to cooking; this is particularly important with poultry.
- Food that has been defrosted should not be re-frozen.

Food handlers

Staff who are food handlers are a potential source of food borne infection. If any member of staff has diarrhoea or vomiting they and their manager must be aware of the potential for cross-infection. Guidance (CDR, 1995) aims to make restrictions simpler to follow, and most people can return to work 48 hours after a formed stool or cessation of vomiting. However if a class one food handler is found to be a carrier of *Salmonella typhi* (Typhoid fever) they cannot work until they are completely cured.

Food handling risk groups

There are risk groups in food handling as follows.

- Food handlers whose work involves touching unwrapped foods to be consumed raw or without further cooking.

- Staff of health care facilities who have direct contact, or contact through serving food, with susceptible patients or persons in whom an intestinal infection would have particularly serious consequences.
- Children aged less than 5 years of age who attend nurseries, nursery schools, playgroups or other similar groups.
- Older children and adults who may find it difficult to implement good standards of personal hygiene – for example, those with learning disabilities. Any guidelines for the exclusion of infected individuals in the last two risk groups assume that they may return once they have passed a normal stool and can subsequently practise good hygiene under supervision. If this is not the case, individual circumstances must be assessed.

Outbreaks of foodborne illness

Food poisoning was defined in 1992 as 'any disease of an infectious or toxic nature caused by or thought to be caused by the consumption of food or water' (CDR, 1995). Food poisoning is obviously a very serious problem, whether it occurs in someone's own home, a restaurant, a hospital, school or nursing home. All potential outbreaks should be investigated by the Environmental Health Department (Department of Health Working Groups, 1994). The investigation of all outbreaks, including foodborne illness is described in Chapter 13.

Laundry arrangements

The laundry service in a hospital, residential or nursing home is often something that is taken very much for granted by staff, but rarely thought about unless there is a shortage of linen. It is generally expected that all used linen is adequately decontaminated before it is used again.

Linen, meaning all articles which require laundering, falls into three different categories under HSG(95)18 (NHS Executive, 1995).

- *Used (soiled and foul)*
  This includes all used linen, irrespective of its state. It can on occasion include linen contaminated with blood and body fluids.

- *Infected*
  This is all linen from patients who are known to or are suspected of having an infection such as dysentery, hepatitis A, B and C, salmonella infections, open pulmonary tuberculosis, HIV, or other notifiable diseases.

  Any linen suspected of being from someone suffering from an infection, such as a viral haemorrhagic fever, must have their linen steam sterilised prior to laundering.

- *Heat labile*
  These include fabrics that will be damaged by the normal heat disinfection process (65°C).

Segregation and decontamination

The different categories are segregated and decontaminated in the following ways.

- *Used*
  For transportation, the linen should be placed in white or off white bags. The washing process should have a disinfection cycle in which the temperature in the load is maintained at 65°C for not less than 10 minutes, or preferrably 71°C for not less than three minutes.

- *Infected*
  Linen in this category should not be sorted by the laundry workers. Immediately after use, the linen should be placed in a red water-soluble bag which is itself in a red outer bag. Once the bag arrives at the laundry, the outer bag will be taken off and the water-soluble inner bag, together with its contents put, directly into the washing machine.
      The temperatures are as for used linen, however there is still some controversy surrounding the inactivation of hepatitis B virus (HSG(95)18), but it is felt that the heat inactivation at these temperatures and the dilution factor should render the laundry safe to handle after the final wash.

- *Heat labile*
  It is advisable not to use these fabrics where possible. However, if they are washed they will need to be washed at low temperatures, which will not disinfect the linen.

These categories do not follow universal precautions, when all blood and body fluids are seen as potentially dangerous. HSG(95)18 states that it is up to the local hospital infection control committee to interpret these guidelines, deciding what should fall into the category of used and infected linens.

Some hospitals have decided that all linen that is covered with blood or body fluids is infected, others will only class blood as potentially infectious, and others will only class blood or body fluids from a known infectious patient as infected.

In the UK nearly all hospital laundry is now sent out to commercial companies (DoH, 1988) who collect used linen and supply rented linen, theatre apparel and bed clothes to the hospital. This means that hospitals no longer have their own laundries or 'own' their own linen. Correct decontamination of linen is vital as the potential for cross-infection to many different hospitals is enormous.

In nursing and residential homes, laundry tends to be done on the premises. Staff will segregate the linen and wash most at 65°C. They will also do their own ironing.

Laundry workers, whether working in a large commercial laundry or at home, should wear appropriate protective clothing, and have a follow-up system in case they suffer from a sharps injury from a needle/scapel hidden in the laundry.

REFERENCES

Ayliffe, G.A.J. (1994) Clinical Waste: how dangerous is it? Current Opinion in Infectious Disease. *Current Science*, **7**, 499–502.

British Medical Association (1990) *A Code of Practice for the Safe Use and Disposal of Sharps*, BMA Professional Division, London.

British Standards Institute (1990) *Specification for Sharps Containers BS7320*, BSI, London and Milton Keynes.

Carlise, D. (1989) Ensuring safe practice. *Nursing Standard*, **3** (41), 25–7.

CDR (1995) A working party of the PHLS Salmonella Committee. The prevention of human transmission of gastrointestinal infections, infestations and bacterial intoxications. A guide for public health physicians and environmental health officers in England and Wales. *CDR*, **5** (11), R158–72.

Daschner, F.D. (1993) The Hospital and Pollution: Role of the Hospital Epidemiologist in Protecting the Environment, in *Prevention and Control of Nosocomial Infections* (ed. R. Wenzel), Williams and Wilkins, Baltimore, pp 993–1000.

Department of Health (1988) *Competitive Tendering in the Provision of Domestic, Catering and Laundry Services*, EL(88)MB/171, DoH, London.

Department of Health Working Group (1994) *Management of outbreaks of foodborne illness*, BAPS, DoH, London.

Gibbs, J. (1991) Clinical Waste Disposal in the Community. *Nursing Times*, **87** (2), 40–1.

Griffiths, G. (1989) Safety in Disposal. *Nursing Standard*, **4** (8), 52–6.

Health and Safety Commission (1992) *The Safe Disposal of Clinical Waste*, HMSO, London.

Health Services Commission (1994) *The Control of Substances Hazardous to Health Regulations*, HMSO, London.

HSE (1985) *Reporting of Injuries, Disease and Dangerous Occurrences Regulations (RIDDOR)*, HMSO, London.

HMSO (1974) *The Health & Safety at Work Act (1974)*, Chapter 37, HMSO, London.

HMSO (1989) *Control of Pollution Amendment Act (1989)*, Registration of Carriers, Chapter 14, HMSO, London.

HMSO (1990) *Environment Protection Act (1990)*, HMSO, London.

HMSO (1991) *Waste Management: Duty of Care (1991), A Code of Practice*, HMSO, London.

HMSO (1992) *Controlled Waste Regulations Stat. Instrument 588*, HMSO, London.

Howarth, G. (1994) All wrapped up, *Greenhouse*. Issue 1, Inst Health Sciences, Oxford.

Muir Grey, J.A. (1994) Greening the NHS: 1989–1994. *Greenhouse*, Issue 1, Inst. Health Sciences, Oxford.

NHS Executive (1995) *Hospital Laundry Arrangements for Used and Infected Linen*, HSG(95)18, HMSO, London.

Renger, M. (1993) EC Waste Law: Regulating the EC Waste Mountain. *Environment Information Bulletin*, 17 March, 1993, 7–8.

Royal College of Nursing (1994) *Disposal of Health Care Waste in the Community*, RCN, London.

FURTHER READING

Barrie, D. (1994) Infection Control in Practice. How hospital linen and laundry services are provided. *Journal of Hospital Infection*, **27**, 219–35.

DHSS (1994) NHS Estates. Health Building Note 25 – Laundry. *Guidance on layout of laundries and segregation of linen. DHSS Tech. Rep. EEL(94)13*.

DoE (1994) Clinical Waste Management. Paper 25. *Department of the Environment Tech. Rep.*

London Waste Regulation Authority (1994) *Guidelines for the segregation, handling and transport of clinical waste*, London Waste Regulation Authority, London.

NHS (1992) Management of Food Services and Food Hygiene in the NHS. *NHS Tech. Rep. HSG(92)34*.

Immunisation

12

Immunisation is the process of artificially stimulating the production of antibodies that protect against invasive disease. Immunity can be induced through active or passive methods, against a wide variety of bacterial and viral pathogens.

ACTIVE IMMUNITY

Active immunity involves the injection of potent antigens that stimulate the immune system to produce antibodies, and depends on stimulating an immune response similar to that which occurs after natural infection. The first recorded vaccine was developed in China almost 1000 years ago (against smallpox). However, Edward Jenner pioneered the scientific basis of the practice in the 1790s, protecting against smallpox by injecting a related cowpox virus. Almost a century later, the work of Koch and Pasteur on cholera, anthrax and rabies brought immunisation into the modern era, leading to the potential to control a range of previous killer diseases.

Today, active immunisation is induced by using two main types of vaccines:

- killed or inactivated vaccines;
- live attenuated vaccines.

Killed or inactivated vaccines

There are three types of killed or inactivated vaccines.

- Supensions of killed organisms such, as inactivated (Salk) poliovaccine or Pol/Vac (intact), typhoid and whooping cough vaccines.
- Components of organisms such as influenza, meningococcal and pneumococcal vaccines.
- Toxoids, which are altered toxins detoxicated by formalin, as in diphtheria and tetanus toxoids.

Live attenuated vaccines

There are two main types of live vaccine.

- A strain of the living organism attenuated so that it loses its disease producing capacity but retains its ability to promote antibody formation, such as tuberculosis vaccine (BCG), measles, oral poliovaccine (Sabin) or Pol/Vac (oral), mumps and rubella vaccine.
- A related organism which produces immunity but little or no disease, such as the vaccinia virus which was used in the vaccination against smallpox.

Most vaccines depend for their action on the production of a serum antibody response (IgG), and by priming the specific immunologic memory. Some, for example poliomyelitis, also lead to the development of local immunity which inhibits invasion of wild virus in the gut. Others, such as BCG, work by stimulating cell mediated immunity.

PASSIVE IMMUNITY

Passive immunity consists of injecting concentrated antibodies, often obtained though concentrating pooled plasma from blood donors (human immunoglobulin). It provides immediate protection but only for the lifespan of the injected antibodies, which may be weeks or months. Passive immunity occurs naturally, such as in the passive transfer of maternal antibodies across the placental barrier in the last 10 weeks or so of the pregnancy. Immunoglobulins are of two types.

- Human normal immunoglobulin, prepared from large donor pools, used for hepatitis A and in the treatment of congenital disorders of gamma globulin production.
- Human specific immunoglobulins made from plasma of selected donors with high antibody levels against particular diseases, e.g. human tetanus immunoglobulin and human rabies immunoglobulin.

THE IMPACT OF IMMUNISATION

Immunisation is notable because it has had a major impact on health in a very short period of time. Smallpox has been eradicated globally, and in the developed world there has been the virtual elimination of diphtheria, tetanus and polio.

In the UK, record low levels of disease notification and deaths from measles and pertussis are the direct result of increased levels of herd immunity achieved through mass immunisation programmes. Rubella notifications are also very low, reflecting interruption of transmission from infected children to pregnant women.

Worldwide, the Expanded Programme on Immunisation (EPI) which began in 1977, when the WHO began working with a handful of countries to demonstrate the feasibility of a multiple antigen immunisation programme in the developing world, has progressed to being a truly global operational programme involving most of the countries of the world.

The contribution of immunisation cannot be overestimated. In the absence of immunisation programmes, four out of every 1000 school age children would be paralysed by poliomyelitis. This figure does not include those infected who would die, or those who would recover. Measles, which in 1982 killed about two per 1000 cases in the USA, killed two per 100 cases in the developing world, rising to 10 or more in malnourished populations. Neonatal tetanus in many areas accounted for 20–50% of the total child mortality (EPI, 1982).

The decision to prevent a particular infectious disease by immunisation depends on the balance between the safety and effectiveness of the vaccine and the cost, frequency and severity of the disease. This latter information on the epidemiology of an infectious disease is derived through surveillance programmes, which provide information crucial to the evaluation of existing immunisation programmes, as well as decisions on the utility of developing new vaccines. Such epidemiological information, derived from the surveillance of measles activity, was crucial information for the UK DoH in deciding that a measles programme was prudent to prevent a sharp increase in measles morbidity in unimmunised pockets in 1994.

THE ROUTINE IMMUNISATION SCHEDULE

There has been a routine immunisation schedule for babies and children for many years (Table 12.1). However, immunisation is a rapidly changing field, and the schedule needs to be reviewed regularly. In 1990, a new accelerated vaccine schedule was introduced, immunising children routinely against diphtheria, pertussis and tetanus at two, three and four months of age. This schedule has been shown to lead to a higher uptake of the vaccines at an earlier age, and levels of immunity at school entry have been shown to be satisfactory, although the actual levels of antibody to both tetanus and diphtheria are lower than in those immunised at three, five and nine months, as in the previous schedule.

The childhood vaccines are administered simultaneously as a single injection, and at the same time as oral polio vaccine. On 1 October 1992,

Table 12.1 Routine immunisation schedule

When is the immunisation due?	Which immunisations	Type	Date the immunisation is given
At two months	Polio	By mouth	
	Hib	One injection	
	Diphtheria		
	Tetanus		
	Whooping cough		
At three months	Polio	By mouth	
	Hib	One injection	
	Diphtheria		
	Tetanus		
	Whooping cough		
At four months	Polio	By mouth	
	Hib	One injection	
	Diphtheria		
	Tetanus		
	Whooping cough		
At 12 to 15 months	Measles	One injection	
	Mumps		
	Rubella		
At 3 to 5 years (usually before the child starts school)	Measles	One injection	
	Mumps		
	Rubella		
	Diphtheria	One injection	
	Tetanus		
	Polio	By mouth	
10 to 13 years (sometimes shortly after birth)	Tuberculosis	Skin test plus one injection (BCG) if needed	
School leavers 14 to 19 years	Diphtheria	One injection	
	Tetanus		
	Polio	By mouth	

a new vaccine against *Haemophilus influenzae* type B (HIB) which killed between 1 and 8% of infected children was introduced into the UK schedule. More than 70% of HIB infections occur before two years of age, and to increase the immunogenic response in children of a few months of age, the vaccine is conjugated either to tetanus toxoid in the Act–HIB vaccine or to a non-toxic variant of diphtheria toxin in Hibtiter.

Immunisation against measles, mumps and rubella is now given as a single vaccine (MMR), introduced in 1988, at 15 months of age onwards. There was considerable debate as to whether a second MMR immunisation was necessary, in order to boost antibody levels, and prevent immunity waning in teenage and young adults, thus leaving them vulnerable to infection from wild measles virus at an age when infection leads to more severe complications. In July 1996, the DoH decided to introduce a second MMR immunisation into the childhood schedule at pre-school entry, along with the booster diphtheria/tetanus and polio.

Achieving immunisation uptake targets

Organisational issues are also important in achieving effective childhood immunisation rates, and recently a new general practitioners' contract proposed the achievement of specific targets for childhood immunisation.

Current health care practices have still not achieved the ideal immunisation levels of at least 95%. An important area which needs further attention in the UK is ensuring that all health care providers are aware of the importance of comprehensive immunisation, and that providers utilise all clinical encounters to screen and, when indicated, immunise children.

Vaccination during pregnancy

Because of a theoretical risk of disease in the developing foetus, which has an immature immune system, live attenuated vaccines are not recommended for pregnant women, or those likely to become pregnant within three months of receiving the vaccine. However, the risk of disease must be weighed against the theoretical risk of damage, and both polio and yellow fever can be given to pregnant women who are at substantial risk of exposure to natural infection.

Although pregnancy is a contraindication to receiving rubella vaccine, data on women who were accidentally or inadvertently immunised with rubella vaccine during pregnancy or within three months of conception demonstrate that the risk of teratogenicity from rubella vaccine virus is negligible. Thus, immunisation with rubella vaccine is no longer considered to be a valid reason for recommending termination of pregnancy. Persons immunised with measles, mumps or rubella vaccine do not transmit the vaccine virus to others, so immunisation of children of pregnant women with these agents is not considered to pose any risk to the pregnant mother.

THE SPREAD OF INFECTION

Infection in child care centres

The spread of infection in child centres is facilitated by the young age and increased susceptibility from immature immune systems of the children, their close contact and lack of understanding of personal hygiene, and an environment in which many items of equipment are shared also contribute to the spread of infection.

Studies of the knowledge of infection control practice in day care settings suggest that employees do not always understand how infections are transmitted, or have the knowledge to prevent or control those diseases common to day centres. Few day care centres provide in service education programmes to their staff on infection control (Smith, 1986). In these circumstances complete immunisation of children attending child care centres is particularly important in reducing the transmission of diseases such as measles, rubella, pertussis, polio and diphtheria.

Herd immunity

The prevention of communicable diseases in the child care environment is significantly facilitated as a result of herd immunity in the general population. When a high proportion of the population is immune, the chain of transmission between infected and susceptible persons is much more likely to be broken, because all of those exposed are immune. The precise effect of herd immunity varies from disease to disease. For example, both the carriage and transmission of *Corynebacterium diphtheriae* and *Haemophilus influenzae* are inhibited in immune populations, although the mechanisms are not clearly understood. In contrast, immunisation with pertussis does not appear to affect circulation levels of the wild bacteria (Fine and Clarkson, 1982).

Hospital

All hospitals run the risk of nosocomial infections – that is infections *acquired* in the hospital, as well as infections that are brought into the hospital. Historically, perhaps because of their focus on acute care issues, infection control practices in the acute hospital environment have failed to maximise the role of vaccines, whose effects are more obvious when considered over a longer time span than the average length of inpatient stay.

In practice, vaccines have a critical role to play in the prevention of a number of severe diseases within the hospital environment.

Hepatitis B

Hepatitis B can infect liver cells and result in both acute and chronic hepatitis. Health care workers (HCWs) can be infected by injury from a sharp object contaminated with blood, splashing of blood or blood stained body fluids onto the eyes or mucosa, or as the result of being bitten by a patient who is a carrier. While almost one third of those infected have an asymptomatic illness, another third suffer serious symptoms of vomiting, abdominal pain, and jaundice. About 1% will develop a fulminant hepatitis, from which most will die within 10 days from liver failure.

Depending very much on the age at infection, some individuals will fail to clear the virus and become chronic carriers. About 50% of these persons are at risk of developing chronic and serious liver damage, including cancer in later life.

A vaccine for protection against hepatitis B has been available since 1982, and it is extremely safe and highly protective. Despite a campaign by the British Medical Association, since 1987, national guidelines were not published until August 1993, HSG(93)40, partially prompted by continuing outbreaks of hepatitis B caused by infected healthcare workers transmitting infection to patients in their care. This 1993 guidance recommended that:

> ''e' antigen carriers must not carry out exposure prone procedures, that is procedures where there is a risk that injury to themselves will result in their blood contaminating a patient's open tissues.'

More importantly, it placed a clear responsibility on employers to ensure compliance with the guidelines that all health care workers performing exposure prone procedures, as well as medical, dental, nursing and midwifery students should be immunised, and that their response to the vaccine should subsequently be checked. It drew attention to the need for employers to comply with Health and Safety legislation by undertaking a risk assessment for all HCWs, and offering immunisation as appropriate.

Tuberculosis

The strategy for control of tuberculosis in the UK has developed around the use of BCG vaccine. BCG vaccine is not a single entity, but has been derived from different strains of the tubercle bacillus which have been passaged many times to produce a less virulent *Mycobacterium*. National guidance, issued in 1994, recommended that all health care workers should be protected against tuberculosis by BCG immunisation.

Varicella (chickenpox)

Chickenpox is a highly contagious disease that in children usually produces a mild illness, but in adults, the immunocompromised and pregnant women can cause more serious disease, and these groups are at higher risk of complications. Nosocomial transmission of varicella is well recognised, and airborne transmission in hospitals has been demonstrated when varicella has occurred in susceptible persons who have had no direct contact with the index case (Leclair *et al.*, 1980).

Many hospitals, particularly those dealing with a high proportion of immunocompromised patients, undertake serological screening of their HCWs. Vaccine is now recommended in the USA for all HCWs who are susceptible (MMWR 1996), and available data indicate that the risk of transmission of vaccine virus to susceptible persons appears to be minimal. Use of the vaccine is also recommended for post exposure immunisation of exposed susceptible persons but, as the efficacy of the vaccine in this situation is still uncertain, such persons should be managed as unvaccinated persons.

The hospital environment also provides health encounters appropriate for opportunistic immunisation. Such opportunities occur in the accident and emergency department, and paediatric and care of the elderly services. The immunisation status of patients should be routinely checked, and those who are susceptible offered immunisation.

Nursing homes and residential homes

Largely due to concerns surrounding the care of patients colonised with MRSA, there has been an increasing recognition of the need for general infection control guidelines for nursing and residential homes. The Public Health Medicine Environmental Group (PHMEG), and Department of Health published *Guidelines on the Control of Infection in Residential and Nursing Homes*, (DoH/PHMEG 1996).

As persons share both eating and living accommodation, there is a very real possibility of infection spreading in a residential establishment. Many such residents will have factors that predispose them to an increased risk of infection, including old age, poor personal hygiene, incontinence and general debility.

In this environment, food safety is paramount, and nursing and residential homes should pay strict attention to food hygiene, to ensure that any risk of infection is minimised. Specific foods may require special precaution in the elderly, and include: shell eggs, which should be thoroughly cooked to avoid *Salmonella enteritidis* infection; paté and soft ripened cheeses, both of which have been identified as important vehicles for *Listeria*, to which elderly persons or those who have impaired immunity are particularly vulnerable.

Immunisation provides added protection against infection, and all homes should have in place an accurate method of maintaining immunisation records on each resident and on all staff. Apart from ensuring that all routine immunisations have been received, that is diphtheria, polio and tetanus, the two most important diseases in residents of homes for which immunisation is available and should be used, are pneumococcal infection and influenza. Although the recommendations in the UK are to immunise only those in higher risk groups with serious chest, heart or kidney disease with pneumococcal vaccine, evidence from the USA demonstrates clearly that there are important benefits to be gained through having a comprehensive immunisation programme in these areas. The UK guidance recommends influenza immunisation for all those living in residential and nursing homes.

Residential accomodation for the mentally ill

A higher prevalence of hepatitis B carriage has been found among certain groups of the mentally ill living in residential accommodation than in the general population. One contributing factor to this is that infection with hepatitis B in persons with Down's syndrome commonly leads to a chronic carrier state. Such persons once infected thus remain an important source of infection, and are more likely than the general population to reside in some form of sheltered accommodation. It is therefore recommended that all staff and the clients of residential accommodation for the mentally ill are immunised against hepatitis B.

Vaccines for travel

The decision to prevent a particular disease by immunisation rests on an assessment of the risks of infection and the efficacy, side effects and costs of the vaccine. The risk is influenced by both the length of the traveller's stay, and the activities once in the foreign country. The only vaccine for which there is a legal requirement is yellow fever vaccine when travelling in the endemic yellow fever areas of Africa and South America. There are certain vaccines that are probably still overprescribed. For example, the vaccine available for cholera is of low efficacy, and is not recommended for protection.

Typhoid should always be given to those travelling to the Indian subcontinent, where most cases identified in the UK originate. Rabies is a serious disease, endemic in many countries and the vaccine is highly effective. Protection can however also be given by post exposure prophylaxis, slightly reducing the need for routine pre-exposure immunisation.

For persons visiting endemic areas where they will be away from urban areas, e.g. backpacking, pre-exposure immunisation is recommended. For those holidaymakers who will only be staying in the larger towns it is unnecessary, although any exposure should be taken seriously. While most exposures will be obvious, special care is needed when visiting areas frequented by bats. A significant proportion of recent cases reported from the USA with virus variants associated with bats have occurred without an unequivocal history of bite exposure.

Smallpox eradication – one of the most significant achievements in the history of public health, demonstrated the enormous cost effectiveness of disease control programmes. Since the last case of smallpox was detected in Somalia in 1977, the world has saved $20 billion.

Individual vaccines

BCG (bacille Calmett–Guérin)

The role of BCG vaccine in tuberculosis control strategies varies markedly from country to country; some, such as the USA, limit the use of BCG vaccine to specific high risk situations, in particular to infants and children in whom the likelihood of *Mycobacterium tuberculosis* transmission and subsequent infection is high. In the UK on the other hand, BCG has, since its introduction for general use in 1953, been a major component of the prevention strategy, and has been routinely offered to schoolchildren between the ages of 10 and 13 years, and in many parts of the UK there is also a programme of immunising newborn babies at risk.

Much of the uncertainty about the value of BCG results from the widely varying results obtained from vaccine field trials. Reported rates of efficacy have varied widely. Most vaccine studies have been restricted to newborn babies or children, and rates have varied from zero to 80%. The largest community based trial was conducted from 1968 to 1971 in southern India. Although two vaccine strains, considered to be the most potent were used, no protective efficacy was demonstrated in either adults or children five years later. Re-evaluation 15 years after BCG was introduced showed that protective efficacy in persons immunised as children was 17%; no protective effect was noted in persons immunised as adolescents or adults.

BCG is not a single vaccine, and many different BCG vaccines are available worldwide. Some of the reported variations in efficacy probably arise from variations in the vaccine itself. Two meta-analyses of reported vaccine efficacies confirmed that the protective efficacy of BCG for preventing serious complications of TB in children is high (>80%), but did not clarify the protective efficacy of BCG in adolescents and adults. The first of these studies reviewed data from 10 randomised clinical trials and eight case control studies published since 1950 (Rodrigues *et al.*, 1993). It showed a greater than 80% protection against meningitis and miliary tuberculosis in both clinical trials and the case control studies. The second meta-analysis reviewed 14 clinical trials and 12 case control studies (Colditz *et al.*, 1994) and showed that protective efficacy was overall 51%, and protection was greater in those immunised as children rather than those immunised at a later age.

Current recommendations are to continue with the school programme and immunisation at birth to those born into high risk groups, which includes babies born to immigrants from high risk countries.

Diphtheria

Diphtheria affects the upper respiratory tract and more rarely the skin. The *Corynebacterium diphtheriae* produces a toxin which affects both cardiac and nervous tissues.

The introduction of immunisation in 1940 has resulted in a dramatic reduction of cases from 46 281 in 1940 to a situation where endemic carriage has been eliminated, with the few cases identified in the last 10 years in the UK almost entirely originating from infection acquired abroad.

Diphtheria immunisation results in the production of a protective antitoxin. It is routinely given in a combined preparation along with polio and pertussis vaccines, and the course consists of three doses separated by one month intervals. A specific low dose diphtheria vaccine preparation is available for use in all persons over the age of 10 years for both primary immunisation and for boosting antibody levels in persons who have been exposed.

Hepatitis B

Hepatitis B virus causes an inflammatory disease of the liver, and is known to be transmitted from one person to another by exposure to infected blood or other body fluids including semen, vaginal fluid and saliva. It has been estimated that 60–80% of newborn children and 6–10% of adults who become infected will become chronic carriers. Such chronic infection can have serious health consequences, including cancer of the liver. HBV kills approximately 1.5 million people each year worldwide (Maynard *et al.*, 1989).

The modern hepatitis B vaccine (HBV) is a non-infectious vaccine which contains purified protein particles from HBV grown in a culture of genetically engineered yeast cells, and it is referred to as recombinant DNA hepatitis B vaccine. The hepatitis B vaccine that was prepared from pooled human plasma is no longer available in the UK.

Approximately 96% of persons immunised will develop a protective antibody response, following a course of three intramuscular injections into the deltoid muscle.

Hepatitis B infection is considered to be the major infectious occupational hazard for healthcare workers. Although effective vaccines have been available for 10 years, and repeated recommendations have been made for the vaccination of health care workers, immunisation rates in North America and Western Europe have been at or below 50% for several years (McCloy, 1993).

Arbitrary schedules for immunisation vary, but are usually 0, 1 and 6 months, or 0, 1, 2 and 12 months. An anti-HBs titre of $> 10iu/l$ is regarded as being protective, although some prefer to see a level of $> 100iu/l$ to ensure there is good protection. Levels of antibody fall progressively with time. It should be noted that increasing age, male sex and smoking all act to reduce the peak antibody levels reached (Cockcroft *et al.*, 1990).

Much discussion has taken place with regard to the necessity for booster doses, particularly in persons who are exposed continually to a risk of infection. It remains unclear at this time whether a booster dose is necessary. Studies in homosexual men have shown excellent protection for up to seven years against significant aspects of the disease (Hadler, 1988). It should be noted in this regard that there are no reported cases of clinical hepatitis or carrier state in persons who have been immunised successfully ($> 10iu/l$ anti-HBs) in up to 10 years follow-up, despite the loss of antibody in many individuals. However, it is known that some individuals do develop anti-HBc, indicating that infection has occurred, even though no illness occurs. What seems to happen in these individuals is that immunological memory induces a rapid anamnestic response in individuals who are subsequently exposed.

In the UK, employers are now required to ensure that all health care workers who perform exposure prone (invasive) procedures are immunised against HBV. This also includes independent contractors, such as general practitioners and dental surgeons working outside the hospital setting, as well as medical, dental, nursing and midwifery students. Those determined as HBe–Ag carriers must have their work restricted.

HBV legislation

The need for a European Community (EC) policy on hepatitis B prevention at work has been recognised for a long time. Despite independent legislation in Belgium, France, Switzerland, Spain and Luxembourg, and national recommendations in the UK, Greece and Portugal, the elimination of HBV as an occupational infection has not succeeded. A general framework directive concerning various risks in the workplace, but not specific to HBV, was agreed in 1989 and came into force in 1993.

Until recently only the Biological Agents Directive, adopted in

November 1990, was more directly related to hepatitis B. This and a more recent directive (NHS Management Executive, 1993) covers the general protection of workers from risks related to exposure to biological hazards. However, it did not address the specific issue of HBV or other vaccine preventable disease. On 6 February 1993, the European Parliament adopted a resolution calling for the immunisation of health care workers and others in 'at risk' occupations, against hepatitis B. An amended version was formally adopted by the Council of Ministers on 12 October 1993. This amended code of practice should have been in place in each member state since April 1994.

Under this code, all EC employers will have to perform a risk assessment of their workers to identify those at risk of being exposed to any virus or bacteria. If exposure to biological agents is confirmed, and effective vaccines exist, the employers must explain the risk and offer immunisation to their workers.

It should be noted that, although hepatitis B immunisation of all health care workers is now in place, and is becoming part of the routine work of the occupational health programme, other types of hepatitis, for example C, have now been recognised. Although they are not apparently as infectious as hepatitis B, they are a reminder yet again of the value of an infection policy based on a concept of universal infection control precautions (Chapter 9).

Influenza vaccine

Influenza viruses are classified according to whether they are type A or B, and by possession of one of two surface antigens – H (three subtypes) and N (two subtypes). Infection with a virus of one subtype provides little or no protection against another, and because over time, changes in the surface antigens can be so great, previous infection with the same strain many years previously may no longer provide protection. For this reason, a review of prevalent subtypes is undertaken every year to help predict the antigenic strains which will be included in that year's influenza vaccine. Usually the vaccine will contain two type A strains and one type B strain.

When an influenza epidemic occurs, rates of hospitalisation of persons in the high risk groups increase markedly, and there is a corresponding rise in death rate. Because the proportion of elderly persons in the UK is increasing, and because age is a risk factor for severe influenza illness, deaths from influenza are also likely to increase unless more active measures to prevent infection are implemented.

Most vaccinated children and adults develop high protective antibody titres, which provide good protection against strains closely related to the vaccine strain. However, the elderly, and persons with a chronic disease, mount a poorer response to the vaccine. Even in such poor responders the vaccine may limit the severity of the attack, and can be effective in preventing superimposed upper respiratory tract infection.

If the vaccine provides a good match to the circulating strains, efficacy approaches 70%. Even though the efficacy in the frail, elderly residents of a nursing home may be much lower, often in the region of 30–40%, they remain 80% effective in preventing death among this population. This is partly because achieving a high rate of immunisation in nursing home residents can reduce the spread of infection through herd immunity.

Certain groups are considered to be at higher than normal risk from influenza infection, and are targeted for vaccination efforts. These groups include:

- persons >65 yrs of age;
- residents of nursing and residential homes;
- persons with chronic respiratory disorders;
- individuals suffering from chronic metabolic diseases, renal dysfunction, haemoglobinopathies and immunosuppression.

In the USA, but not in the UK, groups that can transmit influenza to persons considered to be at high risk are also recommended for immunisation. These persons include:

- health care workers in the hospital and outpatient settings;
- employees of nursing and residential homes who have contact with the residents;
- providers of home care to persons at risk;
- household members – including children – of persons in high risk groups.

Pneumococcal vaccine

Streptococcus pneumoniae is the bacteria which causes pneumococcal invasive disease, and it is an encapsulated bacteria, of which 84 capsular types have now been characterised. Fortunately, only approximately 10 capsular types are responsible for some two thirds of invasive disease in children and about 85% of disease in adults.

Invasive pneumococcal disease is common, especially among the very young and the elderly, and those with underlying medical conditions including immune impairment. In the UK, pneumococcal pneumonia affects approximately 1 in 1000 adults every year, with a mortality of 10–20%, and it is the commonest cause of community acquired pneumonia. Case fatality rates vary by age, but for some high risk patients, have been reported to be as high as 40% for bacteraemia and 55% for meningitis, despite appropriate antibiotic therapy (CDC, 1989).

Pneumococcal vaccine has been available since 1983 as a polyvalent vaccine containing 23 capsular type pneumococcis which together account for about 90% of all pneumococcal disease. In the last decade, high level drug resistant (penicillin and multi-drug) strains of the bacteria have increased substantially and, as with most respiratory pathogens, where the diagnosis is presumptive, the choice of antibiotic for therapy is empiric. In these circumstances, as with all bacteria which show multi resistance, preventive therapy becomes increasingly important. As drug resistance increases, the benefits of an effective immunisation campaign will become increasingly obvious, and markedly more cost effective.

Polio

Polio is a disease that was universally feared as little as 40 years ago. It has been successfully controlled in industrial countries through the development of effective vaccines and large scale immunisation programmes. For those who have grown up in the last 40 years, polio is now a forgotten disease.

In 1988, the World Health Assembly established a target to eradicate poliomyelitis worldwide by the year 2000. The reported global incidence of polio fell to 6179 in 1995, the lowest figure ever and an 82% decline from cases reported in 1988 when the target was set, and a total of 150 countries reported zero cases. The two major areas where polio eradication still needs to be intensified are parts of the Indian subcontinent and Central and Western Africa, as endemic and epidemic outbreaks still continue to occur.

The polio virus exists as one of three types (I, II, and III). Infection may be clinically asymptomatic, produce a non-paralytic fever or result in an aseptic meningitis or permanent paralysis. The ratio of inapparent infections to paralytic disease may be as high as 1000 to 1 in young children.

The first vaccine used was the Salk inactivated vaccine in 1956, which was replaced in the UK by oral attenuated live virus vaccine in 1962, which is always given by mouth. The vaccine contains strains of all three wild types, and produces antibodies in the gut cells. These antibodies provide local resistance of invasion of wild virus, and the net effect is to reduce the amount of wild virus circulating in the community. The vaccine strain of virus may persist in the faeces for up to six weeks.

Primary immunisation is carried out as part of the routine childhood immunisation programme at two, three and four months of age. It is important to note that breast feeding is not a contraindication, and does not reduce the antibody levels produced.

The prolonged excretion of vaccine virus can and does lead to infection of contacts. Such infection is equivalent to immunisation, and may lead to protection of unimmunised individuals. However, in susceptible adults exposed in this way cases of paralytic polio, although extremely rare, have been reported. In England and Wales there has been an average of one recipient and one contact case every year in relation to over two million doses of oral vaccine. Unimmunised adults should be immunised at the same time as their children. There is no need to boost immunised adults, as the exposure to virus excreted by the child itself acts as a booster dose. In families where there is an immunocompromised child, inactivated polio virus is available and should also be used for the siblings and other household contacts.

For the primary immunisation of adults, a course of three doses of oral polio vaccine at intervals of one month provides long lasting immunity. Booster doses after a complete primary course are unnecessary unless persons are at special risk such as:

- travel to an endemic or epidemic area;
- health care workers in contact with a case of poliomyelitis.

For persons at risk, a reinforcing dose should be given every 10 years.

After a single case of paralytic poliomyelitis following infection by wild virus, a dose of OPV should be given to all contacts, irrespective of their immunisation history. When laboratory confirmation is obtained that the index case of polio is secondary to vaccine virus, no immunisation of contacts is necessary, as no outbreaks due to vaccine virus have been reported.

Tetanus vaccine

Tetanus disease is induced by the toxin of the tetanus bacilli which grow anaerobically at the site of an injury. It is characterised by the development of muscular rigidity, and has an incubation period which ranges from 4 to 20 days, usually about 10 days.

Immunisation against tetanus is achieved with a vaccine that protects by stimulating the production of an antitoxin. A cell free concentration of toxin is first treated with formaldehyde, which converts it into the immunogenic but harmless toxoid. On its own the toxoid is not very immunogenic, and to increase its ability to stimulate antitoxin it is usually combined with an aluminium salt.

Primary immunisation is usually given as a component of the childhood immunisation programme as a single vaccine containing diphtheria and tetanus toxoids and pertussis (DPT), at two, three and four months of age. A booster dose of diphtheria and tetanus is given at school entry, and a further reinforcing dose of tetanus at school leaving age.

For older children and adults, primary immunisation is achieved with three intramuscular doses of 0.5ml vaccine spaced at least one month apart. It is now believed that a booster dose 10 years after the primary course is completed, repeated again 10 years later provides sufficient immune response to provide lifelong immunity. Further doses are not required, unless an injury occurs.

Local reactions around the injection site of pain, redness and swelling may occur and last for a few days. Systemic reactions, such as headaches, malaise, fever and muscle pain are uncommon. Acute anaphylactic reactions have been reported, but are rare complications.

Vaccine–drug–vaccine interactions

Information regarding vaccine–drug interaction is important to prevent harm to patients during well intentioned interventions. Knowledge of vaccine–vaccine interactions are important for public health planners who have only limited opportunities for vaccine delivery to susceptible populations.

The safety of routine simultaneous administration of mumps–measles–rubella (MMR) with booster doses of diphtheria and tetanus toxoids with pertussis vaccine, and trivalent oral polio vaccine have been confirmed (Deforst *et al.*, 1988).

Some interactions, such as that between antitubercular drugs and BCG, which impair the immune response to BCG, are well established. Others, such as the interaction of chloroquine and intradermal human diploid cell rabies vaccine, when a decreased immune response is seen in persons concurrently taking long term prophylaxis with chloroquine are less well known. However, they have important practical consequences, i.e. rabies immunisation should be completed at least one month before malaria prophylaxis is commenced. Similarly, an interaction between hepatitis B and yellow fever vaccine has been reported (Yvonnet *et al.*, 1986). This has importance in those countries where hepatitis B is common, or in travellers to yellow fever endemic zones, where doses should be separated by one month if possible.

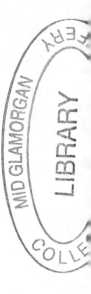

REFERENCES

Centers for Disease Control (CDC) (1989) Pneumococcal polysaccharide vaccine. *MMWR*, **38**, 64–7; 68–77.

Cockroft, A., Soper, P., Insall, C., *et al.* (1990) Antibody response after hepatitis B immunisation in a group of health care workers. *Brit. J. Ind. Med.*, **47**,199–202.

Colditz, G.A., Brewer, T.F., Berkey, C.S., *et al.* (1994) Efficacy of BCG vaccines in the prevention of tuberculosis: meta-analysis of the published literature. *JAMA*, **271**, 698–702.

Deforst, A., Long, S.S., Lischner, H.W. *et al.* (1988) Simultaneous administration of measles–mumps–rubella vaccine with booster doses of diphtheria–tetanus–pertussis and poliovirus vaccines. *Paediatrics*, **81**, 237–46.

DoH/PHMEG (1996) *Guidelines on the Control of Infection in Residential and Nursing Homes*, HMSO, London.

Expanded Programme on Immunisation (1982) *WER*, **57**, 249–56.

Fine, P.E.M. and Clarkson, J.A. (1982) The recurrence of whooping cough; possible implications for assessment of vaccine efficacy. *Lancet*, **ii**, 666–9.

Hadler, S. (1988) Are booster doses of hepatitis B vaccine necessary? *Ann. Int. Med.*, **108**, 457–8.

Leclair, J.M., Zaia, J.A., Levine, M.J. *et al.* (1980) Airborne transmission of chickenpox in a hospital. *New England Journal of Medicine*, **302**, 450–3.

Maynard, J.E., Kane, M.A. and Hadler, S.C. (1989) Global control of hepatitis B through vaccination: role of hepatitis B vaccine in the expanded programme on immunisation. *Rev. Inf. Dis.*, **11** (S3), S574–8.

McCloy, E. (1993) VHPB position on defining and assessing the risk of hepatitis B, in *Procedures of the International Congress on Hepatitis B as an Occupational Hazard* (eds J. Hallauer, M. Kane, and E. McCloy), 1–12 March 1993, Vienna. London VHPB – Medical Imprint 1993. *Tech. Rep.*

MMWR (1996) Prevention of Varicella, *MMWR*, **45**, No. RR–11.

NHS Management Executive (1993) Protecting health care workers and patients from hepatitis B virus. Recommendations of the Advisory Group on Hepatitis, HSG(93)40. *Tech. Rep.*

Rodrigues, L.C., Diwan, V.K. and Wheeler, J.G. (1993) Protective effect of BCG against tuberculous meningitis and miliary tuberculosis: a meta-analysis. *International Journal of Epidemiology*, **22**, 1154–8.

Smith, D.P. (1986) Common day care diseases; patterns and their prevention. *Paediatric Nursing*, **12** (3), 178–9.

Yvonnet, B., Courdaget, P., Deubel, V. *et al.* (1986) Simultaneous administration of hepatitis B and yellow fever vaccines. *Dev. Biol. Stand.*, **65**, 205–7.

Outbreak control | 13

Outbreaks of infection are extremely costly in terms of inpatient care (DoH, 1995), morbidity and mortality. A study undertaken in 1980 (Meers et al., 1980) of HAI in England and Wales showed that 20% of all hospital inpatients had an infection, half of these infections are acquired in the community and half in the hospital. A more recent study undertaken in 1993/94 in the UK and Republic of Ireland reported the prevalence of hospital inpatients with an HAI to be 9.0% (Emmerson et al., 1996). This means, that on average, 10% of all inpatients in a hospital have acquired an infection since their admission. Prevalence rates of HAI are higher in teaching hospitals (11.2%) than in non-teaching hospitals (8.4%) (Emmerson et al., 1996). The most common infections are urinary tract infections (23%), lower respiratory tract (23%), surgical wound infections (11%) and skin infections (10%). These figures show that despite, or maybe as a result of the medical advances in the twentieth century, hospital infection is still commonplace, a fact that most health care workers appreciate, but that few patients and the general public do.

A strategic infection control programme properly financed and including trained infection control personnel has been shown to reduce the incidence of HAI (Haley, 1985). Part of this programme is a system for preventing outbreaks of infection in the hospital, and also having a plan if such an outbreak does occur.

Outbreaks of infection do occur in the community, and can have enormous consequences (Editorial, CDR, 1990) though to date there is no community equivalent of the hospital infection control document. Local authorities have outbreak plans, and most hospital outbreak plans have a section to include the community.

THE COST OF HOSPITAL INFECTION

The cost of HAI in the UK has been estimated at between £1000 to £2000 per patient (DoH, 1995). The true cost of HAI is undoubtedly far greater.

The health service reforms have brought about a great many changes in trust finance, and outbreak costs can be divided into two; costs directly attributed to outbreaks and opportunity costs.

Costs directly attributed to outbreaks

- More expensive nursing care, physiotherapy, occupational therapy, etc. as caring for patients in isolation takes extra time. One system of controlling outbreaks is cohort nursing, which means that staff may be segregated between looking after known infected patients and others who are not known to be infected. In practice this means that agency and locum staff are generally employed to care for patients not known to be infected. This can have a large impact on staff costs.
- Moving beds around during outbreaks may result in less flexibility in staff deployment and therefore creates the need for more agency staff.
- Drugs that are used may be more expensive, particularly if the outbreak is caused by an organism that is resistant to the normally used first line cheaper drugs. Thus, treating the cause of the outbreak will mean using expensive drugs.
- Any additional specimen taking increases the amount of staff time on the wards to actually take the specimens and increases the costs in the laboratories to process the specimens.
- If patients stay in hospital longer than expected they cost more in terms of bed days.
- Costs from the supplies department for gloves, aprons, etc. may rise.
- Domestic staff may have to clean the ward or department more often.

In many hospitals, if multi-drug resistant organisms (e.g. MRSA) have continued to rise steadily for a number of years, this will usually be taken into consideration in the hospital accounting, and these expected costs will be met in the annual budget. Unexpected costs arising from outbreaks will however not be met in the year's budget, so expense will have to come from another source.

Hospital accounting systems are not yet sophisticated enough to reflect the true costs of outbreaks in all budgets, so that even though, for example, physiotherapists may have had costs due to an outbreak this will in no way be reflected in their allocated budget.

Opportunity costs

Trusts can suffer severe financial loss if they do not use beds and operating theatres efficiently. These losses can be minimal under block contracts with large tolerances on the contract volumes. However, block contracts of little or zero tolerance may result in trusts reimbursing marginal costs to health authorities where activity has not met contract targets. Another very important factor is the increasing number of GP fundholders, well over 50% nationally. Many fundholders now have block contracts, but many procedures are still paid for on a cost per case or cost and volume basis. This means that cancelling GP fundholder patients can lead to the loss of full cost income rather than just marginal cost. This also applies to any emergency contract referral income.

These opportunity costs, associated with patient cancellations if a hospital has an outbreak and cannot operate on patients on the waiting list, can have very significant cost implications for trusts, i.e. at 1996 prices many hundreds of thousands of pounds a year. The reason the costs are so high is that areas with high costs such as orthopaedics, vascular surgery and oncology are also the areas where patients are particularly at risk from infection. If there is an outbreak, infection control teams tend to close these areas to admissions quickly to prevent infections in implants, transplants and patients who are already severely immuno-compromised.

The increase in day surgery over the past decade has resulted in many more dependent patients being admitted as inpatients than in the mid-1980s, which means that a ward in the 1990s has far more susceptible patients undergoing higher cost invasive procedures than previously. If there is an outbreak, these people cannot be sent home as they are too ill, neither can many of the operations be cancelled as they may be deemed as life threatening. Controlling outbreaks in these areas relies heavily on the use of risk assessment, the expertise of the infection control team and the judgement of clinical staff. In areas such as an intensive care unit the decision to close the unit to admissions cannot be taken lightly as people may be at more risk of dying because the unit is shut rather than the associated morbidity or mortality of a nosocomial infection. It is important to state that not all hospital acquired infection is preventable, and neither is it likely to become so in the foreseeable future.

OUTBREAKS OF INFECTION IN HOSPITAL

It is generally accepted that hospital inpatients are more susceptible to infection than the general population. With the increasing number of people being discharged from hospital earlier, many people in their own homes, hospices, nursing and residential homes are increasingly susceptible to infection. Susceptibility to infection is affected by age, by pre-existing disease and by the medical, surgical or immunosuppressive treatment the patient receives. Many infections are caused by the normal commensal organisms which people carry on their bodies. Invasive procedures in hospitals provide a route by which these normally harmless organisms can invade the body and cause an infection.

Although most cases (90%) (DoH, 1995) of infection are not recognised as outbreaks, even preventing an outbreak can have cost implications. It is difficult to calculate the cost benefits of preventing or controlling outbreaks, however this form of infection control will probably save money in the long term. In the USA (Haley, 1985), it has been estimated that investing in an infection control team, with one full time infection control nurse, a part time infection control doctor and a secretary for every 250 beds, will be repaid if infections are reduced by 6%.

Arrangements for the control of outbreaks in hospital

Outbreaks of infection in the hospital may vary between just a few cases of, for example, surgical wound infection to very large outbreaks, such as if there is an outbreak of food poisoning. It is the responsibility of the hospital infection control team, together with the CCDC to draw up detailed outbreak plans appropriate to the local situation (DoH, 1995). These plans should go through the hospital ICC and be ratified formally. The plans must be clearly written, detailing how to convene an outbreak control group (OCG) and when and how such a group will become a major outbreak control group (MOCG).

Role of the CCDC and ICD in outbreaks

Since 1988, CsCDC have been in existence to give valuable advice to both the hospitals and the community. They have expertise in the diseases most commonly causing outbreaks in the community. However, many of the organisms which cause outbreaks in hospitals, such as MRSA, *Klebsiella*, and vancomycin resistant enterococci (VRE), fall within the level of expertise of the ICD and medical microbiologist. The CCDC does have valuable epidemiological knowledge which he can use in these situations. It is therefore very important, even during small hospital outbreaks, that the CCDC is always informed, and that the ICD and CCDC agree to work together during outbreaks to utilise their skills to the greatest benefit of everyone concerned.

It is very important for one person to be designated to take the lead during outbreaks and this should be written clearly into the hospital outbreak plan.

Recognising outbreaks

Small outbreaks of infection occur in hospitals on a frequent basis, and tend to comprise part of the regular routine of the hospital ICT. However small or insignificant an outbreak may seem, it is vitally important that the ICT do meet formally to discuss the outbreak and that a report is produced. An outbreak may be suspected through a number of ways:

- health care workers on a ward or in a department may notice an increase in infection rates, or be concerned that they think there may be a problem;
- the microbiological laboratory reports may show an increase in the isolates of a single species from one particular area;
- the occupational health department may notice an increase in the incidence of infection in staff;
- diseases that are statutorily notifiable to the proper officer of the local authority (usually the CCDC) may lead to recognition of an outbreak.

Rapid recognition of an outbreak is vitally important. For this to occur there should be good liaison between the ICT and others working in the hospital. It is important that all staff feel that they can mention the possibility of an outbreak to the ICT and know that their feelings will be taken seriously. Routine surveillance of infection may help to identify infections, however some outbreaks may occur very slowly, and may sometimes have almost finished before they are recognised.

Investigating a potential outbreak

In hospital the person primarily responsible for taking action, in the event of a potential outbreak, is the ICD. The ICD and ICN will take the appropriate action to determine whether an outbreak exists or not and this should not normally take more than a couple of hours. At the end of this period the severity of the outbreak should be assessed and some immediate control measures put in place. If the ICT have investigated a suspected outbreak and found that none exists they need to reassure staff and patients while, at the same time, ensuring that any future reporting is not discouraged.

If the ICT believe that there is an outbreak they need to:

- determine if the outbreak may be a major outbreak;
- determine if there is the possibility for community involvement.

Outbreak control

Each hospital should have an outbreak plan which should outline the action to be taken depending on the nature of the outbreak.

Objectives of an outbreak plan

- To ensure prompt action.
- To determine the course of the outbreak.

- To prevent further spread.
- To prevent recurrence.
- To ensure all necessary agencies are informed promptly of a possible outbreak.

To achieve this it is essential to have an outbreak plan which is based on the following principles:

- all staff should be made aware of the definition of an outbreak;
- all staff must know who to inform if they suspect an outbreak;
- all staff should be familiar with the normal infection control policies in place in their health care setting;
- the outbreak plan should be reviewed yearly;
- good communication networks should be established.

Limited hospital outbreak

For a small hospital outbreak a meeting of the Outbreak Control Group (OCG) will normally need to be called. The OCG will consist of:

- the ICT, and secretarial support;
- the chief executive or his representative;
- the CCDC;
- a nurse or midwife representative from the area affected;
- clinicians from the area affected.

The functions of OCG:
- To review the evidence and decide whether there really is an outbreak.
- To develop a strategy for dealing with the outbreak and allocate responsibility for action to members of the OCG who are then accountable for ensuring that action takes place.
- To control the spread of the disease by implementing appropriate control strategies.
- To provide an accurate and responsible source of information for other health care workers, the media and public.
- To produce reports.

It is the responsibility of the ICT to present information on the outbreak, its history, and predictions for the future to the OCG and to produce draft plans and guidance for future management of the outbreak. If the outbreak is small and well managed the OCG may not need to meet again, and the CCDC may not wish to be part of the OCG. A formal report of the outbreak should be prepared by the ICT, circulated to the OCG and the hospital infection control committee (HICC). This report should be discussed at the next HICC meeting.

In some areas the members of the district infection control committee have endorsed a standard report form for all ICTs to complete following an outbreak. This form contains the following information:

- members of ICT:
- date outbreak first reported;
- where outbreak reported, hospital and ward, etc;
- specialty of ward/department;
- dates of onset, signs and symptoms of outbreak, microbiological reports;
- date OCG meeting called, or if not reason why;
- brief summary of meeting(s) and recommendations, e.g. ward closed to admission;
- date outbreak declared over;
- recommendations;
- costings to ICT.

Outbreaks not confined to hospital

In these outbreaks, or where more than one hospital is involved, the CCDC is the person primarily responsible for all procedures outside the hospital. However, an OCG should still be called. Health authorities and local authorities should have outbreak polices in place for community outbreaks (DoH, 1995).

MAJOR OUTBREAKS

All outbreak plans should include a definition of what constitutes a major outbreak. The definition will depend on a number of factors, the number of people concerned, the pathogenicity of the organism concerned and the potential for spread in the hospital and/or community. If the ICD in a hospital sets in place the major outbreak plan, the CCDC will as the proper officer to the local authority inform the chief medical officer. The CCDC is also the person who has the responsibility to communicate and as appropriate consult with the CDSC.

Major Outbreak Control Group

If a major outbreak control group is called (MOCG) additional members to the smaller OCG will be:

- additional hospital management;
- medical director;
- executive nurse director;
- an infectious diseases expert;

- occupational health department representative;
- director of public health;
- chief environmental health officer if there is a possibility that the outbreak is food or water borne;
- director of PHLS;
- regional epidemiologist.

In some situations, additional expertise may be needed, this could include:

- consultant virologist;
- CSSD manager;
- pharmacist;
- catering manager.

Functions of the MOCG

When an outbreak has been identified the functions of the MOCG are:

- to ensure that the clinical care of the patients involved in the outbreak is not compromised;
- to ensure there are adequate resources, both human and in terms of equipment;
- to ensure that all members of the MOCG are sure of their roles, and that functions are carried out by specific individuals who are responsible for that action;
- to ensure good communication between all members of the MOCG, other hospital staff, outside experts and the media;
- to meet frequently, normally daily;
- to define the end of the outbreak;
- to prepare a preliminary report, and a final report.

OUTBREAKS IN THE COMMUNITY

Outbreaks may also occur in nursing or residential homes or other care establishments in the community. In these situations, it is normally the community infection control nurse and CCDC who will do the initial investigations to ascertain whether an outbreak is occurring or not. The CCDC may call an OCG which will consist of:

- CCDC;
- CICN;
- relevant general practitioner(s);
- manager/owner of the establishment;
- registration officer;

- environmental health officer, if there is the possibility that the outbreak is food or water borne;
- relatives;
- others specific to that area of work.

It is the responsibility of the CCDC and CICN to present information on the outbreak, its history, and predictions for the future to the OCG and to produce draft plans and guidance for future management of the outbreak. If the outbreak is small and well managed the OCG may not need to meet again. A formal report of the outbreak should be prepared by the CCDC and CICN, circulated to the OCG and discussed at the next district infection control committee (DICC).

Major outbreak in the community

As with the hospital, there may be times when the CCDC will suspect a major outbreak. This may be due to food borne illness or another communicable disease. In the case of food borne illness, guidance (DoH, 1994) is available. Food poisoning has been defined in this guidance as 'any disease of an infectious or toxic nature caused by or thought to be caused by the consumption of food or water'.

In this situation, the CCDC will convene a major outbreak control group which may include the following in addition to the people on the OCG:

- director of public health;
- medical microbiologist;
- occupational health representative;
- ambulance services;
- chief environmental health officer;
- water company representatives;
- regional epidemiologist;
- representative from the CDSC.

Functions of the MOCG:

- To ensure that the care of any individuals involved in the outbreak is not compromised.
- To ensure there are adequate resources, both human and in terms of equipment.
- To ensure that all members of the MOCG are sure of their roles, and that functions are carried out by specific individuals who are responsible for that action.
- Ensure good communication between all members of the MOCG, other hospital staff, outside experts and the media.

- To meet frequently, normally daily, to review systematically the situation.
- To define the end of the outbreak.
- To prepare a preliminary report, and a final report.

At the end of the outbreak, once it has been controlled, the MOCG should meet one more time with the following objectives:

- to declare the outbreak over;
- to review the experience of all participants involved in the management of the outbreak;
- to identify any shortfall or particular difficulties that were encountered;
- to revise the outbreak plan if necessary;
- to make recommendations for structural or procedural improvements which would reduce the chance of occurrence of the outbreak.

REFERENCES

Department of Health (1995). *Hospital Infection Control; guidance on the control of infection in hospitals* (Prepared by the Hospital Infection Working Group of the Department of Health and Public Health Laboratory Service), BAPS, Lancashire.

Department of Health Working Group (1994) *Management of outbreaks of foodborne illness*, BAPS, Lancashire.

Editorial CDR (1990) Cryptosporidium in water supplies: the second Badenoch report. *CDR*, **5** (46), 245.

Emmerson, A.M., Enstone, J.E., Griffin, M., Kelsey, M.C. and Smyth, E.T.M. (1996) The second national prevalence survey of infection in hospitals – overview of the results. *Journal of Hospital Infection*, **32**, 175–90.

Haley, R.W., Culver, D.H., White, J.W., *et al.* (1985) The efficacy of infection surveillance and control programs in preventing nosocomial infection in US hospitals. *American Journal of Epidemology*, **121**, 182.

Meers, P.D., Aycliffe, G.A.J., Emmerson, A.M., *et al.* (1981) Report on the National Prevalence Survey of Infection in Hospitals 1980. *Journal of Hospital Infection*, supplement 2.

Infections due to protozoa, helminths, the human louse, and *Sarcoptes scabiei*

14

This chapter discusses infections which emphasise the wider implications of infection control in the community. Some of these infections do cause a considerable amount of ill health and morbidity, while others cause severe disease. Many, such as head lice or thread worm cause minimal ill health but give rise to fears and stigma. Obviously, when ill health results, these infections may be seen in hospitals. Frequently, however, they occur in patients as a secondary diagnosis requiring prompt treatment.

Helminth and protozoal infections emphasise the part man's relationship with animals, domestic or otherwise, can play in the transmission of infection. Control relies on the good working relationships between environmental health officers (EHOs), the Ministry of Agriculture Fisheries and Food (MAFF), and local veterinarians. Liaison and inter-agency work is also required to control outbreaks of scabies or head lice and to deal with cases of crab or body lice. Sadly, even in the latter part of the twentieth century, much of the work involves dispelling myth and allaying fears before control measures can be commenced.

The increase in airline travel since the 1970s, immigration and political unrest, resulting in population movement means that many tropical infections caused by helminths and protozoa may be seen in the UK today. These are not discussed in this chapter. However, whenever a person is unwell, one of the key questions should always be about travel history.

PROTOZOA

The characteristics of the protozoa include the following:

- they are unicellular;
- seen only under the microscope;
- contain a nucleus;
- reproduce asexually in the host;
- may also reproduce sexually in a second host, often in a cystic form.

Some protozoa seen in this country include:

- *Cryptosporidium* spp. causing cryptosporidiosis;
- *Toxoplasma gondii* causing toxoplasmosis;
- *Trichomonas* spp. causing trichomoniasis;
- *Pneumocystis carinii* causing pneumocystis carinii pneumonia (PCP) (Jeffrey and Leach, 1991).

Cryptosporidium

Cryptosporidium is an intracellular protozoan parasite first described in 1907, which remained rare and insignificant for 50 years (Mandel *et al.*, 1995). It was linked to human gastrointestinal illness in the 1970s; in the early 1980s it was linked with diarrhoea in people with acquired immuno-deficiency syndrome (AIDS) and interest increased dramatically. *Cryptosporidium* is recognised as a cause of diarrhoeal illness, and it is probably one of the most common enteric pathogens in humans and domesticated animals worldwide. It may also cause bilary tract and respiratory disease as well.

In humans, the major symptom of cryptosporidiosis is diarrhoea with stomach cramps. Sometimes the infected person shows no signs or there may be fever and nausea. In individuals with a normal immune system it is a self limiting disease but for those who are immunocompromised, particularly with AIDS, severe diarrhoea can persist and be a cause of death. The absence of any reliable or definitive therapy increases the magnitude and significance of cryptosporidiosis.

The sexual cycle of the organism results in the production of oocysts which are passed into the faeces of affected humans or animals. Outside the body they remain infective for two to six months in a moist environment. They can be passed from person to person and animal to person by the faecal–oral route, and via infected water supplies. Outbreaks associated with infected water supplies result in a need to issue 'boil water' orders by the local water authority in conjunction with the local environmental health and public health departments. There is a need for this because chemical disinfection of the water does not destroy oocysts.

Other general infection control measures to prevent spread include careful handwashing after toileting, care when handling animal excreta, e.g. during gardening and cleaning cat litter trays, and handwashing for those involved in the handling of calves and lambs with diarrhoea. Many nursery schools and play groups visit farms as part of the general education of the children, and advice should be given to these groups as outlined below.

Outside visits

This information applies particularly to venues where children have contact with animals. Visits of children to farms, etc. can carry a small but real risk of children acquiring infections particularly gastroenteritis. The main routes of infection being:

- hand to mouth;
- close contact with animals such as lambs/calves.

Prior to the visit teachers/organisers should enquire about the following:

- toilet and washing facilities;
- provision of a separate eating area for picnics etc;
- provision on farm site for isolating sick animals from visitors;
- provisions to prevent curious children sampling animal feed and raw milk;
- general standard of cleanliness in the area to be visited by the children.

During the visit:

- children should be discouraged from putting fingers in their mouths;
- hands must be washed before eating;
- animal food stuffs/raw milk must not be sampled;
- water should be taken from taps marked specifically 'drinking water';
- hands must be washed after close animal contact – discourage children from putting faces close to animals;
- alternative facilities for eating must be found if existing facilities are found to be inadequate.

Toxoplasma gondii

Toxoplasma is an intracellular protozoan which is a major cause of serious infections of humans and domesticated animals. Frequently infection remains asymptomatic. When there are symptoms these include persistent fever and swollen glands. It is a dangerous infection in immunocompromised patients, and people with AIDS frequently have serious infection which involves the brain, muscles or respiratory systems. In early pregnancy infection can lead to intrauterine death or severe birth defects.

Cats, birds and domesticated animals serve as reservoirs. Cats are the definitive hosts as they become infected by eating infected rodents or birds. All other infected animals such as pigs, sheep and chickens are secondary hosts; they carry *Toxoplasma gondii* encysted in muscle or brain tissue. Humans become infected by:

- eating undercooked meat;
- direct contact with cat litter, and failure to wash hands afterwards;
- children via playground contact contaminated with cat faeces (such as in sandpits).

It is not passed directly from person to person, except across the placenta. Prevention is most important in seronegative pregnant women and in immunodeficient patients. However, it is important to remember that seropositive individuals may become infected again. Prevention of infection is easily accomplished. The goal is to avoid ingestion of and contact with cysts or sporulated oocysts. Cysts in meat are made non-infectious by heating the meat to 66°C, by smoking or curing it, or by freezing it to 20°C (which is not possible in most home freezers). Meat should not be eaten rare. Hands should be washed thoroughly after handling raw meat or vegetables, eggs should not be eaten raw, and unpasteurised milk (particularly milk from goats) should be avoided. Vectors such as flies and cockroaches should be controlled.

Cat faeces should be avoided, and gloves should be worn while disposing of cat litter, gardening, or cleaning a child's sandpit. Oocysts are killed if the cat litter tray is soaked in nearly boiling water for five minutes. If the tray is cleaned every day, oocysts do not have a chance to sporulate.

Preventative action – toxoplasmosis

Responsible pet ownership
To prevent toxoplasmosis, it is essential that pet owners are responsible and ensure the following:

- adequate worming regimens for pets;
- clear litter trays daily;
- clear up in public places after a pet defaecates.

Parents and carers
Anyone responsible for the care of children should:

- cover sand pits to keep out cats;
- prevent toddlers from putting soil in mouths;
- wash hands after handling pets and after outdoor play; before eating;
- wash raw fruit and vegetables carefully.

Pregnant women
Pregnant women should:

- avoid cleaning out litter trays if possible;
- wear gloves when gardening;
- avoid contact with lambing ewes.

In addition everyone should ensure the thorough cooking of meat and avoid the consumption of unpasteurised milk.

Pneumocystis carinii

In the 1960s, *P. carinii* became appreciated as an important cause of pneumonia in immunocompromised people. However, with the development of more safe and effective antimicrobial drugs interest waned. The interest in *P. carinii* has again increased since the 1980s with the rise in incidence of pneumocystosis associated with AIDS. *Pneumocystis carinii* is an organism of low virulence found in the lungs of humans and a variety of animals. Its lifecycles are not really understood (Jeffrey and Leach, 1991, Mandel *et al.*, 1995). In one study 75% of normal individuals were reported to have antibodies to *P. carinii* by the age of four years indicative of an infection not causing actual disease (Benenson, 1990). The organism causes an often fatal pneumonia in certain groups such as premature babies, those chronically ill and the immunocompromised patient. Disease in immunocompromised patients is possibly a reactivation of a latent infection or it may be due to direct transmission (Benenson, 1990). Reactivation can be prevented by the administration of prophylactic drugs. Research is continuing into this organism and effective prevention.

Trichomonas spp.

There is no cystic stage linked to this protozoa. *Trichomonas vaginalis* was first described in the nineteenth century and older literature frequently describes it as a harmless commensal. In women *T. vaginalis* causes vaginitis with small haemorrhagic lesions on the mucous membrane of the genital tract, together with a profuse foul smelling discharge. It can also be asymptomatic. In men it is usually asymptomatic but the organism is present in the prostate and seminal vesicles. It is thought to cause 3% of all non-gonococcal urethritis (Benenson, 1990). It is therefore a common sexually transmitted disease and infection can be passed on over a period of years as infection is present in an asymptomatic patient.

Actual signs of disease are more common in women and control of the infection is by treating cases and their partners, and also by contact tracing and treating any other previous or present partners.

HELMINTHS

The Ebers papyrus dated at 1500 BC described various helminthic diseases (Muller, 1975). Worm infections in humans and other animals constitute a significant contributor to the global burden of illness caused by infectious diseases.

The characteristics of helminths include the following:

- they are multicellular large organisms;
- visible to the eye;
- may measure from 1mm to several metres;
- reproduce sexually in the host;
- have larva and ova stages usually in a second host.

Infection may occur directly via the faecal–oral route when an egg or larvae is swallowed. Alternatively, infection can occur when infected meat, fish or vegetables are eaten. In some cases, the larvae may penetrate the skin, e.g. *Schistosoma* spp.

Worldwide, millions of people are affected by helminth infections. In some areas with malnutrition they cause much morbidity and are an avoidable cause of death (Meers *et al.*, 1994). Only those species likely to be seen in the UK are discussed (Table 14.1).

Table 14.1 Classes of worms

Abroad	UK
Nematodes	
Ancylostoma duodenale (hookworm)	*Enterobius vermicularis* (thread, pin or
Strongyloides stercoralis	seat worm)
(strongyloidiasis)	*Trichinella spiralis* (round worm)
Dracunculus medinerus (Guinea worm)	*Toxocara canis/cati* (toxocariasis)
Cestodes	
Taenia solium (pork tape worm)	
Taenia saginata (beef tape worm)	
Diphyllobothrium latum (fish tape	
worm)	
Echinococcus multilocularis	*Echinococcus multilocularis* (dog tape
(dog tape worm)	worm)
Trematodes	
Schistosoma species (blood flukes)	*Fasciola hepatica* (sheep liver fluke)
Paragonimus westermani (lung fluke)	

Classes of worm

Three are three classes of worm that can infect humans:

- nematodes (round worms);
- cestodes (tape worms);
- trematodes (flukes).

Nematodes

Enterobius vermicularis (thread, pin or seat worm)
This worm has been described in Greek, Roman, Arabic and Chinese writings from as early as 400 BC (Muller, 1975). It is the most common nematode parasite in developed countries. Children are usually affected and infection causes a great deal of unwarranted anxiety among parents, carers and school teachers considering they cause very little actual disease. The worms are 5–10mm long and the females lay their eggs on the perianal skin. This causes an itch and the person scratches. The host, usually a child, then sucks unwashed fingers and the eggs re-enter the gut (in girls the eggs can also enter the vagina), and bedding and clothes can become infected.

When a case of thread worm is diagnosed the whole family should be treated and in multiple cases in schools, large numbers of people may need to be treated. To facilitate treatment and prevent further cases:

- everyone should use their own towels and face cloths;
- change sheets and night clothes as often as possible;
- vacuum carpets often;
- affected persons should wear pants when sleeping to prevent scratching;
- nails should be clean and short;
- hands should be washed on waking before touching surfaces;
- hands should be washed before eating and after toileting.

Treatment, together with the above measures, should control an outbreak. Strict supervision of young children is needed to ensure adequate handwashing and this is not always available in schools or nurseries. Cleaning contracts may make it difficult to arrange the extra toilet facilities and vacuuming of carpets in sleeping/living areas recommended to control large outbreaks in residential homes.

Trichinella spiralis (round worm)
This round worm affects 50 million people worldwide (Jeffrey and Leach, 1991). The reservoir of infection is found in pigs, dogs, cats, rats, arctic mammals and wild animals. Man is infected by eating raw or poorly cooked meats. However, improved food preparation has reduced the incidence of trichinellosis.

The adult worm develops in the intestine and burrows into the intestinal wall and thus to the systemic circulation. The disease may range from mild infection to serious disease or death. Symptoms include diarrhoea, swollen eye lids, muscle pain due to encystment with a concentration in the muscles and respiratory system. It is not transmitted from person to person but animal hosts remain infected for months. Therefore, good food hygiene practice and regulations relating to the preparation of waste offal for feeding to pigs are of vital importance.

Toxicara cani/cati (toxocariasis)

This organism causes a disease called toxocariasis. It is a common parasite of dogs and cats. Nearly all puppies are infected by their mothers and start to pass eggs in their stools by the time they are four weeks old. The eggs then incubate for one to three weeks before becoming infective. They will then remain infective in the soil for many months. Random soil tests frequently reveal evidence of infection.

Infection occurs after contact with contaminated soil, unwashed hands then transfer the eggs to the mouth. Unwashed vegetables and fruit may also be a mode of transmission. The egg hatches and the larval worm enters the blood stream and circulates. Most children who have the infection do not show any sign of illness and so diagnosis is difficult; the most publicised symptom is loss of vision. Prevention is the same as for toxoplasmosis (p. 176) and depends on responsible pet ownership.

Cestodes

Echinococcus multilocularis (dog tape worm)

This tape worm causes echinococciasis or hydatid disease. The larval cysts are found in the liver and can spread to the lung and brain. The cysts continually grow and form large space-occupying lesions. It is a serious disease and difficult to treat. The *E. multilocularis* is perpetuated in nature by a continuous cycle between rodents, foxes and dogs. The adult worms are passed in faeces.

Human infections occur by ingestion from unwashed hands which may have touched dogs who have been rolling on contaminated land. It is not passed from person to person. Preventative methods include:

• periodic treatment of dogs with antihelminths;
• only keeping the needed number of working dogs on farms;
• not allowing dogs to eat uncooked flesh of rodents or herbivores;
• responsible pet ownership;
• families of cases need to be checked.

Specific treatment may include resection of the cyst or chemotherapy.

Trematodes

Fasciola hepatica (sheep liver fluke)
This is a large trematode which is a natural parasite of sheep, cattle and other animals worldwide. Eggs passed in the faeces develop in water, the larvae enter snails and then produce large numbers of cercariae. Human infection can be acquired by eating uncooked aquatic plants, such as water cress, which is contaminated. In the human intestine, migration to the liver and bile ducts occurs. Obstruction of the bile ducts causes severe pain and jaundice. Generally, treatment by drugs is unsatisfactory (Benenson, 1990). Finding the source of any infection should prevent further cases. Land can be drained properly or chemicals used to eliminate the snails. The public should be made aware of the dangers of eating uncooked aquatic plants taken from areas where sheep and cattle graze.

The sites of helminth and protozoa infections are shown in Figure 14.1.

SCABIES

Scabies is an allergy to the mite *Sarcoptes scabiei*. The mite and the disease scabies have been recognised separately since the time of Aristotle, but it was not until 1687 that the link was established between the mite and the disease. However, at the time few were prepared to accept this and most preferred to blame foul 'humours' for the symptoms of scabies. Finally, in 1868, Hebra published a treatise entitled *On Disease of the Skin Including Exanthemata* which lead to the final acceptance of the link between the mite and the disease (Burgess, 1994).

In developed countries, scabies is a disease where the number of cases rises every 20 to 30 years; it is not clear why this should happen. In developing countries, where treatments are not readily available, the prevalence remains very high. Scabetic mange can also occur in mammals other than humans, and in some animals it can be devastating. However, animals cannot be infected by humans or vice versa (Burgess, 1994).

As with any infestation there are many myths surrounding scabies. The author is grateful to Dr J. Maunder of The Medical Entomology Centre, University of Cambridge for supplying the following information. The scabies mite does not survive away from the body, in the environment or on articles, such as clothing or bedding, as the mite dehydrates rapidly once away from its burrow. Scabies can be passed from an infected person to another via skin contact, often through hand holding contact. Scabies is therefore a disease of affection rather than sexual contact. It may take six to eight weeks for an infected person to develop an antibody response to the mite and to develop a rash and start itching. However they may infect others during this period, and will continue to be infectious once the rash occurs.

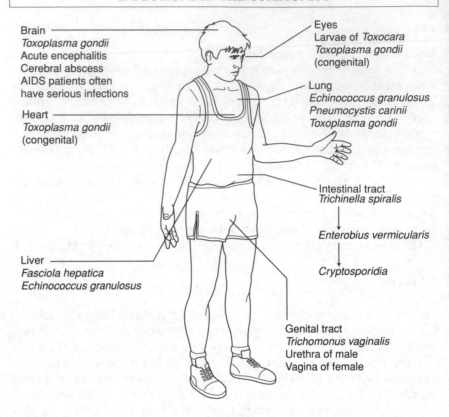

Figure 14.1 Helminths and protozoa: sites of infection (adapted from Muller, 1975, Figure 1)

Sarcoptes scabiei burrow down to the deep layers of the skin where the female lays her eggs which then hatch three days later. At all stages of the life cycle the mites produce faecal pellets which are glued to the tunnel floor. The allergen from these faecal pellets seeps into the deeper parts of the body and into the blood stream so that it is spread all over the body. This systemic involvement of the whole body means that the sites of the allergic reaction, i.e. the rash, do not generally correspond to the sites where the mites may be found. Scabies can present in a variety of ways.

Types of scabies

Classic scabies

This form is found in healthy individuals with normal immune systems. During the first few weeks the mites multiply rapidly, but once the person becomes sensitised, the population reduces to 10 to 20 mites. Most people have no recognisable burrows and this is particularly so in people such as health care workers or food handlers where the skin is softened by frequent handwashing. Burrows may be identified as red, slightly raised papules or vesicles on the wrists, backs of the hands and between the fingers. An absence of burrows does not exclude scabies. Six to eight weeks after the initial infection the person will complain of itching. The rash may be difficult to see but the itching is such that scratching will result in excoriation of the affected areas. Distribution of the rash is characteristic, including the fingers, forearms, axillary folds, sides of the chest, around the waist, lower quadrant of the buttocks, inside the legs and around the ankles. The rash is always symmetrical but may not appear at all sites at once.

Crusted scabies

This was once called Norwegian scabies but this term is no longer used. Crusted scabies occurs in people in whom the immune system is impaired. The itchy rash does not occur but, eventually, areas of scaling and crusting appear anywhere on the body. This form of the disease is highly contagious and it is often at the centre of an outbreak of classic scabies among family members or residents in a nursing or residential home.

Atypical scabies

Classic scabies and crusted scabies are relatively easy to recognise but atypical scabies is an intermediate form. Frequently there is no rash or itching and no scaling or crusting, although the mites may be found anywhere on the body including the head. Certain groups are more susceptible to this form of scabies:

- the very young, i.e. under four years of age;
- people with Down's syndrome;
- the elderly;
- alcoholics;
- people taking immunosuppressive drugs;
- people who are using topical steroids to stop undiagnosed itching;
- people in long-stay institutions.

Diagnosis of scabies

Diagnosis is made by a history of the disease and clinical appearance. Mites choose the site of a skin crease to burrow, therefore it may be possible to identify the mite microscopically from skin scrapings taken from these sites. The presence of a symmetrical rash on the body together with itching which is worse at night is suggestive of scabies.

A scabicide should be used to treat scabies. The development of resistance must always be considered and therefore a mosaic pattern of treatment should be recommended when treating large numbers of people such as in a hospice, nursing or residential home. In addition further treatments may be required for people with symptoms as the eggs are more resistant than the mites.

Treatment

The available treatments include the following insecticides:

- malathion (Derbac M lotion);
- permethrin (Lyclear dermal cream);
- lindane (Quellada lotion; this is the most toxic).

All of the above should be used as stated in the instructions, and any contraindications noted. In general, aqueous preparations are preferable to alcohol lotions, and lotions give far better coverage than creams. *Infected persons with classic scabies are usually non-infectious immediately after treatment.*

Practical treatment guidelines

- The scabicide should be applied to a cool skin, not after a hot bath.
- The lotion or cream should be applied all over the body with special attention to the hands, groin area, behind the ears, hair lines, umbilicus and axillae.
- The treatment must be left on the skin for the prescribed period of time. It should be reapplied to the hands if they are washed and to the buttocks after nappy changing.
- The head should be treated in:
  - immunocompromised people;
  - very young children;
  - the elderly;
  - cases of crusted scabies;
  - previous treatment failure;
  - those with very sparse hair.

Treatment failure often occurs because people only treat the sites of the rash, not the whole body. After treatment the itching can persist for up to two weeks; this is not an indication of treatment failure and the rash should begin to fade over this period.

Guidelines for the management of a scabies outbreak in an institutional setting

A definite diagnosis must be made, preferably by obtaining skin scrapings for microscopic examination. The extent of the problem can be assessed by questioning staff about recent rashes or undiagnosed itching in both residents and health care workers.

An all inclusive treatment plan aims to treat all symptomatic and asymptomatic residents, staff, and families of affected staff members. Therefore, it is important to educate staff to ensure full compliance and correct application treatments. Close co-operation with general practitioners and other visiting staff will be needed if all concerned are to be treated in a set 24 hour period.

Crusted scabies are often the cause of outbreaks in institutions, such as nursing homes, and they are frequently overlooked and remain a source of infection and reinfection of residents, staff and visitors for a long time (Carslaw, 1975). Infected skin scales can be shed by the person with crusted scabies and reasonable care should be taken with personal clothing and bedding belonging to these people. Health care workers should keep this in perspective; bedding does not need to be destroyed. There is no scientific evidence to prove that bedding or furnishings play a significant part in the transmission of the infection. Also, the high temperatures and dry heat in most nursing or residential homes mean the mites dehydrate and die rapidly (Burgess, 1994).

HUMAN LICE

Lice have been recognised for thousands of years and have been associated with disease for some of that time. Remains of ancient lice and their eggs have been found on mummified bodies from ancient Egypt. Before the invention of the microscope it was thought that lice occurred spontaneously from dirt or even decomposing sweat (Maunder, 1983). This association with dirt still exists today and is the possible reason for the social stigma which continually occurs during outbreaks of lice infection.

It is important to appreciate that lice rapidly dehydrate and die when away from the human body. Clothing lice survive a little longer as they frequently have to move through layers of clothing to feed. Lice only rehydrate by feeding on their host's blood. Lice infections cause illogical reactions among communities, which in turn leads to a conspiracy of silence among infected families and a fear of stigma associated with the idea that lice thrive where there is dirt. This conspiracy of silence may prevent adequate treatment of contacts through fear of telling people they are contacts, and may allow for reinfection to occur thus perpetuating outbreaks.

Diseases associated with lice infection

- Impetigo; the role of the louse in the transmission of this infection was first demonstrated in 1892.
- Typhus; mainly transmitted by clothing lice.
- Louse borne relapsing fever; seen in Ethiopia during the famine of the 1980s (Burgess, 1995).

Human lice have not been shown to transmit any type of virus including the human immunodeficiency virus despite speculation in the popular press (Zuckerman, 1986; Taplin and Meinking, 1986).

In the past, treatment relied on physically combing the lice out of the hair or picking them out from clothing. This continues to be the norm in countries where money is not available to purchase treatments. Treatments other than insecticides are becoming increasingly favoured by environmentalists in developed countries, and by those concerned about exposure to chemical treatments. With these treatments, the combing out of lice must continue until all live lice have been removed. Whether most people have the time to do this properly is debatable. Chemical treatments plus limited combing offer a quick solution which many prefer.

Species of lice associated with man

There are three species of lice associated with humans.

- Clothing louse – *Pediculus humanus humanus*
- Crab louse – *Phthirus pubis*
- Head louse – *Pediculus humanus capitis*

Lice infection causes a general allergic reaction to the saliva injected into the site of the bite and this allergic reaction results in itching and a raised area around the site of the bite. In particular, reactions to the prolonged biting of the body louse can give rise to a general illness, lassitude, stiffness of muscles, and a rash all over the body, hence the expression 'feeling lousy'.

The clothing louse

In affluent countries, clothing lice have been virtually eliminated, but are still found where there is poverty, over crowding, homelessness, and upheaval due to civil disturbance.

Persons affected by clothing lice show excoriated skin due to scratching, and the eggs or nits may be seen in the seams of clothes to confirm diagnosis. The clothing louse lives on clothing, especially in the seams and goes onto the body to feed. If the same clothing is worn over a period of time the lice proliferate. The female lays eggs along the seams of the clothes not on the body. The lice are passed to others during close personal contact or by contact with infected clothing or bedding. Infected clothes or bedding become free of lice if they remain unworn or unused for longer than two days (Burgess, 1995). To kill the lice, clothes should be washed at a temperature above 60°C, and tumble drying kills both eggs and lice (Roberts, 1987).

Modern practices of low temperature washes, followed by natural drying and then rewearing the clothes straight away allows any infection to continue. This modern practice emulates practices found during times of war and disaster or severe poverty, i.e. clothing washed in cool water, dried naturally and then immediately reworn.

Summary of the treatment of clothing lice
- A complete change of clothing and bedding.
- Washing at a temperature above 60°C.
- Tumble drying with seams turned inside out.

Shaving the body or bathing the affected person does not achieve anything as the lice live in the clothing, not on the body. Eradication requires political commitment to reduce levels of poverty and homelessness along with financial commitment towards developing countries.

Crab lice

Crab lice are similar to head lice, but their body shape is much flatter and they move more slowly than head lice. They are found in all body hair even eyelashes, not just pubic hair. They may be passed on by sexual contact but physical contact of any type can facilitate transmission. In children they can be passed on by sharing a bed with an infected person, and in the case of babies while breastfeeding. When exposed to light the crab lice becomes less active and therefore less likely to transfer to a new host. They are even less likely to be transferred from contact with objects such as chairs or toilet seats as they dehydrate and die off the body even more rapidly than the head louse (Nuttall, 1918).

Summary of the treatment of crab lice
- Use aqueous based treatments.
- Apply to all hairy parts of the body including the scalp.
- Apply to the eyelashes, if necessary using a cotton wool bud.
- Treat all contacts as transmission occurs socially as well as sexually.

Head lice

Head lice live on head hair and eyebrows. They move all over the scalp so are not more likely to be found at the nape of the neck or behind the ears. Each mature female lays an average of eight eggs a night, sticking each one to the base of the hair shaft next to the scalp where the temperature is optimum for incubation. The eggs resemble the colour of the scalp and so are difficult to see. The eggs hatch in 7–10 days, and the empty egg shell is called a 'nit', as it is white and easy to see. The louse grows by shedding its skin twice before adulthood, and the female becomes capable of reproduction when 10 days old.

Head lice pass from one person to another by crawling across the hairs during prolonged head to head contact. Shared combs, chair backs and hats are unlikely to result in transmission because of the rapid dehydration resulting in death which happens when the louse leaves the body. These shed louse skins sometimes resemble live lice and may give rise to the idea of fomites harbouring lice.

Itching only occurs if the infected person becomes sensitised to the lice saliva. Therefore, the following groups may not present with this symptom:

- those with early infection;
- young pre-school children up to the age of four or five years;
- adults who have had longstanding infections or many infections and are no longer sensitive to lice saliva.

Outbreaks of headlice
Outbreaks of head lice can only be controlled by finding and treating every case.

What to look for:
- six legged insect – match head size;
- live eggs close to the scalp – hard to see;
- empty eggs – nits present on hair shaft away from scalp as the hair grows;
- black/brown dust (droppings) on pillows or collars;
- shed scales on pillows.

N.B. Itching is not always present

How to look:
- use a fine toothed comb or a plastic detector comb from the pharmacist;
- dampen hair;
- part hair in layers and comb;
- live lice may be seen or combed out.

How to treat:
- treatments are available from family doctors or pharmacists;
- everyone should be checked and, when live lice are found, treated;
- continue to recheck hair after treatment;
- comb out dead and dying lice;
- tell everyone who has had close contact with the infected person and ask them to check and treat.

Summary of treatment available for lice
There are various treatments available for headlice, including the following insecticides (brand names in brackets):

- carbaryl – prescription only (Carylderm, Clinicide, Derbac–C, Suleo–C);
- permethrin – (Lyclear);
- malathion – (Derbac–M, Prioderm, Suleo–M);
- phenothrin – (Full Marks).

The shampoo forms of these treatments are not very effective. Also, treatments should not be used as preventatives as this aids the development of resistance.

Non-insecticidal treatments
The theory of these treatments is that they are said to stun, immobilise the lice or dislodge lice and their eggs. They will only be effective if combined with thorough combing of the hair until the lice are removed.

- Ordinary hairwashing – comb out while hair is wet.
- Lavender oil – immerse hair in warm water.
- Tea tree oil – mix with a carrier oil, such as sweet almond oil, massage into the hair and follow by daily rinsing with tea tree oil plus water and combing.
- Lemon juice and vinegar – add to water to wash hair then comb (Roberts, 1987).

Checking for head lice is the responsibility of the individual or parent concerned. In schools, education authority staff do not have the legal right to carry out head inspections and in fact it could be considered as assault. Rarely, school nurses may inspect heads to check if infection is present and recommend treatment. Usually the subject of head lice infections are discussed during pre-school parents' evenings and health promotion sessions are provided on request. Guidelines are produced by the department of public health, education authority and child health department. These designate a particular insecticide for treatment and this is changed every three years to prevent resistance. Circulation of these policies into the wider community is essential as control of head lice remains very much a community responsibility.

REFERENCES

Benenson, A.S. (1990) (ed.) Control of Communicable Diseases in Man, 15th edn, Report of the American Public Health Association. *Tech. Rep.*

Burgess, I. (1994) *Sarcoptes Scabiei* and Scabies. *Advances in Parasitology*, **33**.

Burgess, I. (1995) Human Lice and their management. *Advances in Parasitology*, **36**.

Carslaw, R.W., Dobson, R.M. *et al.* (1975) Mites in the environment: cases of Norwegian scabies. *British Journal of Dermatology*, **93**, 333–7.

Jeffrey, H. and Leach, R. (1991) *Atlas of Medical Helminthology and Protozoology*, 3rd edn, Churchill Livingstone, London.

Maunder, J.W. (1983) The appreciation of lice. *Proceedings of the Royal Institute of Great Britain*, **55**, 1–33.

Meers, P., Sedgewick, J. and Worsley, M. (1994) *The Microbiology and Epidemiology of Infection for Health Science Students*. Chapman & Hall, London.

Mandel, G.L., Bennet, J.E. and Dolin, R. (1995) Principles and Practice of Infectious Diseases. 4th edn, Churchill Livingstone, London.

Muller, R. (1975) *Worms and Disease: A Manual of Medical Heminthology*, London.

Nuttal, C.H.F. (1918) Combatting lousiness among soldiers and civilians. *Parasitology*, **11**, 201–20.

Roberts, C. (1987) A lousy life. *Community Outlook*, August, 1987.

Taplin D. and Meinking, T.L. (1986) Infestations, in *Paediatric Dermatology*, vol. 1.2. Churchill Livingstone, New York, pp. 1465–93.

Zuckerman, A.J. (1986) Acquired immune deficiency syndrome and insects. *British Medical Journal*, **292**, 1094–5.

Infection control in the mortuary

15

Throughout the world many times a day, people are facing one of the most profound of all human experiences, the death of someone they love, and the dying person is faced with their own mortality. The following emotions will be witnessed; anxiety, fear, depression, sadness, denial and acceptance (Kubler Ross, 1982) by people who have contact with the dying and their families.

Therefore, it is essential that a sensitive and sensible approach to the control of infection is taken. A realistic assessment of risk to health care workers (HCWs), carers, relatives and friends must be taken. Of approximately 600 000 deaths per year in the UK, 1% are associated with infection and not all of these actually present an infection risk after death (Young and Healing, 1995).

The relationship between the carers, the dying patient and family is crucial in helping all to understand the need for any additional precautions to prevent the spread of infection. Viewing each patient/client as an individual (Bowell, 1990) allows for individualised care, therefore in infection control, it is possible to reduce precautions to a safe minimum based on research. The principle of universal infection control precautions must be followed after death, as it is not always possible to know if someone was infected in life. This will mean that the patients, relatives and the health care service benefit; the patients because rational explanations can be given for the actions taken, the service because the care is more cost effective.

This individualised approach also allows patients and relatives to understand the nature of any infection and allows discussion about risk to family and friends. This openness is very important if the patient is terminally ill due to an infectious disease; the dying and their family frequently withdraw emotionally from one another (Kubler Ross, 1982); both unable to cope with individual emotions. Fear of spreading infection or alternately contracting an infection may contribute towards or trigger this withdrawal. A study of bereavement support in NHS hospitals in England and Wales in 1988 (Wright *et al.*, 1988) would suggest that professional carers find it difficult to offer compassionate support at the time of relatives witnessing the death of loved ones. Why so many HCWs are unable to provide the emotional support needed during the processes of dying and death is beyond the scope of this book, but if there is an infection element involved, perhaps the carer fears for his or her own health or for the health of their family. Good infection control education should address these fears. In research by Bond (Bond, 1991) and Akinsanya (Akinsanya, 1992) this type of fear featured very prominently among nurses caring for patients with AIDS.

Following death, the risk the body may pose for those who have contact with it is assessed according to the hazard the particular infectious agent may pose. Following death, infections which are both notifiable and non-notifiable under the Public Health (Control of Diseases) Act 1984, and the Public Health (Infectious Diseases) Regulations 1988 may or may not create an infection risk after death. It is possible to assess the risk these organisms may pose by referring to the Advisory Committee on Dangerous Pathogens 1995 document entitled Categorisation of Biological agents according to Hazard and Categories of Containment.

THE HAZARD GROUP CLASSIFICATION OF MICRO-ORGANISMS

There are four hazard group classifications of micro-organisms.

- Group 1. A biological agent unlikely to cause human disease.
- Group 2. A biological agent that can cause human disease and may be a hazard to employees; it is unlikely to spread to the community and there is usually effective prohylaxis or effective treatment available.
- Group 3. A biological agent that can cause severe human disease and presents a serious hazard to employees; it may present a risk of spreading to the community, but there is usually prophylaxis or treatment available.
- Group 4. A biological agent that causes severe human disease and is a serious hazard to employees; it is likely to spread to the community and there is usually no effective prophylaxis or treatment available.

In each of the groups, 'disease' refers to disease caused by infection.

The more common organisms which may present a hazard to people likely to come into contact with a dead body include:

- hepatitis B virus;
- hepatitis B, plus delta virus;
- hepatitis C virus;
- *mycobacterium tuberculosis*.

Less common organisms include:

- *Salmonella* spp.;
- *Staphylococcus aureus*;
- *Streptococcus* spp.;
- human immunodeficiency virus.

Rare organisms include:

- polio viruses;
- *Corynebacterium diptheriae*;
- rabies virus.

Plus all the rare viruses listed under hazard group 4, e.g. Lassa, ebola and Marburg.

All organisms are placed within one of the hazard groups and they form an approved list of biological agents. This list has legal status invoked by the new COSHH 1994 regulations which came into effect in January 1995 (HMSO, 1994). These listings use a framework of criteria as follows.

- Is the organism pathogenic to man?
- Is it a hazard to workers?
- Is it transmissible to the community?
- Is there effective prophylaxis or treatment available?

It is important for staff to realise that each organism is assigned to one of the hazard groups according to the infective hazard they pose for healthy workers and does not take into account:

- a pre-existing disease;
- compromised immunity (to include any break in the integrity of the skin);
- pregnancy;
- effects of any medication taken.

This in itself emphasises the importance of pre-employment questionnaires for staff and the importance of keeping immunisations up to date.

CARE PROCEDURES AFTER DEATH

Most disease-causing organisms die off after death but commensals, particularly anaerobic bacteria, take over the decomposition process. Therefore, the body, whether previously infected or not may be a source of infection. This should be remembered during all care procedures with strict adherence to UICP (Healing *et al.*, 1995). Some hospitals have dispensed with last offices which involve the packing of the body orifices, stating that it is unnecessary especially in coroner's cases and distressing for nurses to perform. The purging of body fluids does occur after death, especially of the stomach and bowel, wounds also leak, and funeral workers often receive bodies which are unpleasant to handle. Peter Speck, a hospital chaplain, writes of convincing reasons why last offices should be performed and states that they are part of sensitive continuing care and not an archaic ritual (Speck, 1992).

Staff or relatives who handle bodies should perform a risk assessment of the procedures they are about to perform and wear the appropriate protective clothing. If there is a chance they will come into contact with blood or body fluids they should be wearing clean disposable gloves and a plastic apron.

Hygienic preparation

Hygienic preparation of the body is defined as cleaning and tidying the body prior to viewing by family and friends. It may be undertaken by the family, nurses, carers or funeral staff depending on the circumstances (Healing et al., 1995).

Religious beliefs and cultural customs, such as those of Muslims and Jews, must be observed and it should never be necessary to restrict the families of the deceased unless a serious hazard exists.

Hygienic preparation is not recommended when certain infections are present and guidance should be sought from the doctor in charge of the case or the consultant in communicable disease control.

Viewing of the body

This is defined as seeing, touching, and spending time with the body (Healing et al., 1995) after death and before final disposal. There are few infectious diseases where such contact would put friends and relatives at risk. Viewing in the hospital is arranged by the mortuary staff or, out of hours, the ward staff. As with hygienic preparation, the presence of certain infections would contraindicate viewing, e.g. viral haemorrhagic fever, anthrax and plague (Philpott–Howard and Casewell, 1994).

Stillbirths

Rubella, syphilis, toxoplasma, cytomegalovirus, parovirus B19 and listeria monocytogenes are the organisms most likely to cause stillbirth (Healing et al., 1995). They may still be present on the body after death. However, basic washing of the body and wrapping in a cloth should reduce any risk of transferring infection to the family who may wish to hold and spend time with the body. The father in particular may have been the source of the infection or exposed to it during the pregnancy, therefore handling the body poses little extra risk.

The use of body bags

There is widespread use of body (cadaver) bags. When body bags are used the rate of cooling of the body is slowed and therefore decomposition occurs more rapidly. Bodies reach the funeral directors in a poor condition and are frequently unfit for hygienic preparation, thus denying the relatives the opportunity to view the body. Policies for the use of body bags should be clearly thought out with the best interests of the relatives, friends, health care staff and funeral workers taken into consideration.

There are circumstances when body bags should be used, and advice should be sought as above. Body bags should be used if the body is thought to present a serious infection risk, e.g. HIV, AIDS, other blood borne viruses and notifiable diseases. In these cases a biohazard label should be attached to the death certificate which is placed on the body bag. If the body is leaking, it is also sensible to place it in a body bag. There are different types of body bags available, some are easier to use than others. When a body bag is used relatives should be encouraged to view the body before the bag is closed.

Once the body bag has been closed the risk of infection is removed and staff do not need to wear any protective clothing when handling the body. This is one of the reasons why many hospitals routinely use body bags, however, staff should wash their hands afterwards.

THE MORTUARY

A mortuary is necessary (Health and Safety Commission, 1991) for various reasons.

- To maintain body tissues in a condition whereby the maximum scientific information can be obtained from the post mortem examination and subsequent analytical investigations.
- To prevent tissue decomposition while burial or cremation arrangements are made.
- To hold bodies and the occasional specimen for longer periods in conditions of security.
- To provide facilities for bodies to be viewed or identified by relatives or friends.
- To carry out post mortem examinations.

Post mortem investigation will always be important in providing coroners with accurate information about sudden cause of death (natural or unnatural), accidents, industrial disease and allegations of medical error or malpractice.

In order to fulfil these functions and, at the same time, provide safe working environments employers and employees, whether in hospital mortuaries or private funeral premises, have obligations under key Health and Safety Legislation (Table 15.1) The legislation, approved codes of practice, working party reports and policy documents provide a framework for good practice in all aspects of mortuary work including infection control.

Structure and design of the mortuary or funeral premises need to comply with certain standards (DoH, 1991), providing non-pervious surfaces which can be easily hosed down and cleaned. There should be designated 'dirty' and 'clean' areas with restriction on entry into the dirty areas by non-designated staff (Health and Safety Commission, 1991). This control of movement extends to relatives, clergy, all personnel attending a post mortem and all personnel collecting or delivering bodies. Everyone should be encouraged to wash their hands thoroughly before leaving the mortuary.

Table 15.1 Some Acts and regulations

Health and Safety at Work Acts, 1974
To ensure the health and safety of all those who may be affected by work activities by providing safe premises, equipment, systems of work, training of staff and a written safety policy [if more than five employees]

Health and Safety First Aid Regulation, 1991
To ensure first aid facilities are available to treat staff and visitors or contractors

Reporting of Injuries Diseases and Dangerous Occurrences Regulations [RIDDOR], 1989
To ensure certain specified accidents and/or work related illnesses are reported to the Health and Safety Executive

Control of Substances Hazardous to Health Regulations, 1988 and 1994
To ensure that substances hazardous to health are identified, risk assessed, adequately controlled, employee health is monitored when appropriate, training is provided about the risk and controls needed.
COSHH, 1994 Implements two European Directives, the second of which contained a European Community classification of biological agents capable of causing infection [93/88/EEC] and provides the basis for the hazard groups discussed in the text. This 1994 regulation also gives legal status to this hazard group listing as an Approved List of biological agents

Management of Health and Safety Regulations, 1992
These regulations overlap with much of the previous legislation and regulation but does tend to be more specific in the areas it covers and more stringent in its requirements in terms of risk assessment, training, etc. It also deals with specific groups of workers in a more detailed way e.g. of pregnant workers

---

The body store should be large enough to cope with anticipated storage requirement of bodies. Storage cabinets should operate at a reduced temperature (approximately 4°C). A separate room for the storage of specimens is required with air extraction ventilation to ensure concentrations of the fixative vapour (i.e. formaldehyde should not exceed two parts per million for any period of exposure).

A dedicated supply and extraction ventilation system is required for the post mortem suite, body storage areas, dirty utility room and staff changing rooms. Ten changes of air per hour are recommended for provision of pleasant working conditions, but this is probably not necessary for the prevention of spread of infection (Babb *et al.*, 1989).

Mortuary staff and staff working in the funeral services are advised to contact their local infection control service about safe working practices as health authority infection control policies may be available for guidance.

Infection control hazards in the mortuary

The most common hazards likely to be encountered with examples of causative organisms are:

- blood borne viruses – HIV and HBV;
- enteric infections – *Salmonella* spp., *Shigella* spp., hepatitis A;
- wound infections – *Streptococcus pyrogenes*, *Staphylococcus aureus*;
- septicaemic infection – *Neisseria meningitidis*;
- respiratory infection – *Mycobacterium tuberculosis*.

Research has shown that bacterial counts in the air of post mortem rooms were low (Newson *et al.*, 1983). Therefore, contact spread presented the greatest hazard with a significant risk of blood borne infections and wound infections being acquired via cuts and puncture wounds (Babb *et al.*, 1989). This particular research highlighted the following:

- the high incidence of glove punctures during post mortems, particularly amongst the technicians;
- the skin of the cadaver was frequently contaminated with Gram-negative bacilli during necroscopy and these numbers were not appreciably reduced after cleaning;
- frequently, hands were heavily contaminated after removal of gloves, emphasising the need for effective handwashing;
- dissection boards and necroscopy tables remained heavily contaminated even after cleaning so disinfection was recommended.

Procedures during a post mortem such as cutting tissue (e.g. lung or incising abscesses) can present a hazard and the sawing of bone could release contaminated chips of bone into the air. The high incidence of glove punctures highlights the risk of sharps injuries from needles, other sharps instruments and ragged bone injuries.

Contaminated aerosols or splashes may be released through squeezing tongues, washing down the body after necroscopy and during the hosing down of surfaces in the post mortem room. Research in America (Johnson and Robinson, 1990) stated that certain procedures used in surgery on bone and soft tissue, i.e. the use of bone saws, could expose personnel to an HIV infection hazard if the resulting aerosols were contaminated, but the joint working party of the Hospital Infection Society Study Group (Shanson, 1992) has discounted this mode of transmission and feel the American research methods were flawed.

Researchers took air samples while cranial saws and band saws were used and, despite the fact that large numbers of tracer organisms were applied to bone, few were recovered during or immediately after the use of the saw (Babb *et al.*, 1989).

The potential for injury to personnel by sharps highlights the importance of safe working procedures, risk reducing procedures and the importance of having a policy and procedure should such an injury occur.

The Duty of Care, an approved code of practice (Department of Environment, 1991), sets out the individual's responsibilities with regard to the safe disposal of sharps and other clinical waste to prevent injury and cross infection. The Environmental Protection Act, 1990, legislates for the disposal of all types of hazardous waste. Most waste originating in the mortuary can be defined as clinical waste and should be incinerated.

The post mortem room equipment and instruments present a severe challenge to all disinfectants and sterilisation procedures. Most disinfectants are capable of eliminating Gram-positive and Gram-negative bacteria, also enveloped viruses (hydrophobic viruses). Less easily eliminated targets are non-enveloped viruses (hydrophyllic viruses), mycobacteria, particularly atypical, protozoal cysts and bacterial spores.

For equipment and linen the use of elevated temperatures are preferred to the use of chemicals. Contaminated linen and clothing should be placed in alginate bags to avoid the necessity of handling clothing at the laundry and then washed in a hot water wash HSG (95) 18 (HMSO, 1995). For equipment, the use of elevated temperatures to sterilise is preferred. For unwrapped instruments the minimum temperature/time for sterilisation is 134–138°C for three minutes. If a hot water boiler is used there must be immersion in boiling water (98–100°C) for a minimum of five minutes. It is recommended that every mortuary should have a hot water boiler steriliser (HSC, 1991). Careful decontamination of instruments prior to chemical or heat sterilisation is necessary.

Two types of aldehydes (formalin, 10% solution of formaldehyde, and glutaraldehyde 2%) are found in post mortem rooms. As with all such chemicals, COSHH regulations must be followed when using them. Formalin is used to perfuse suspected tuberculous lung tissue and for fixing fresh histological material. Glutaraldehyde is used for disinfection. Neither are suitable for environmental decontamination.

Summary of infection control practice in the mortuary

Measures to prevent the spread of infection in the mortuary and post mortem room can be summarised as follows.

Primary prevention
- Good communication between the following:
  - general practitioner and mortuary/funeral service staff;
  - wards and mortuary staff;
  - mortuary staff and the funeral services.
- Correct and proper training of all workers.
- The provision of a safe working environment.
- Good working practices.
- The correct use, dilution and storage of disinfectants.
- Effective decontamination procedures.

Secondary prevention
- Immunisation and staff health surveillance.
- The correct use of protective clothing and equipment.
- Correct ventilation system.
- Personal hygiene to include hand washing procedures.

Tertiary prevention
- Safe, correct disposal of clinical waste.
- Security and restricting access to the mortuary area.
- Care and supervision of visitors and observers.

FOLLOWING A DEATH, WHO IS AT RISK?

Hospital and community

- Construction workers.
- Archaeologists.
- Doctors and pathologists.
- Nurses and midwives.
- Mortuary assistants.

- Forensic scientists.
- Embalmers.
- Funeral directors.
- Emergency services.

Situations where personnel may be particularly at risk

- Old internments.
- Post mortem rooms.
- Attending accidents (Healing *et al.*, 1995).

COMMUNITY ISSUES AND THE FUNERAL SERVICE

Old Internments

Death in previous centuries was mainly due to infection. Some diseases are unlikely to survive burial, e.g. plague, cholera, typhoid and tuberculosis. However, in anthrax and smallpox, survival is possible, the greatest danger is to workers in enclosed places such as crypts. By 1840 over 50 000 corpses were interred in the London area each year in only 218 acres of land, resulting in multiple graves, poor earth covering and frequently a foul smell in the churchyard. The same occurred elsewhere in the UK, and is the reason why human remains are often found on building sites, in towns and cities. Whenever old soft tissue is seen in a damaged or opened coffin there could be an infection risk and the local consultant in communicable disease control should be contacted for advice.

The Funeral services

The hazards which face funeral directors and embalmers are similar to those of mortuary workers but of a lesser order. Funeral directors need information from medical personnel to make the correct decision about hygienic preparation, viewing and embalming of the body. At present, few areas issue infection control guidelines designed specifically for the funeral service. A publication entitled *Health and Safety in the Funeral Service* (Co-operative Funeral Services Managers' Association, British Institute of Embalmers, National Association of Funeral Directors, British Institute of Funeral Directors, 1992) attempts to clarify the situation for funeral directors by providing information based on the assumption that it is not always possible to know when a body may be infected: therefore, for practical purposes the information is based on UICPs.

REFERENCES

Akinsanya, J. (1992) Who will care? A survey of the knowledge and attitudes of hospital nurses to people with HIV/AIDS. *Journal of Advanced Nursing*, **17**; 400–1.

Babb, J.R., Hall, A.J., Marlin, R. and Ayliffe, G.A.F. (1989) Bacteriological sampling of post mortem rooms. *Journal of Clinical Pathology*, **42**, 682–88.

Bond, S. (1991) Experience and preparation of community nursing staff for work associated with HIV infection and AIDS. *Social Science Medicine*, **32**, (1), 71–6.

Bowell, E. (1990) *Infection Control in the Nursing Process. Infection Control Guidelines for Nursing Care*, (eds) M. Worsley, K. Ward and L. Parler, ICNA/ Sugikos, London.

Cooperative Funeral Services Managers' Association (1992) *Health and Safety in the Funeral Service*, John Horbury and Associates, London.

Department of the Environment (1991) *The Duty of Care (ACOP) Waste Management*, HMSO, London.

Department of Health (1991) *Mortuary and post Mortem, Health Building Note 20*, HMSO, London.

Healing, T., Hoffman, P. and Young, S. (1995) The infection hazards of human cadavers. *Communicable Disease Report*, PHLS, **5**, Review 5.

Health and Safety Commission (1991) *Safe working and prevention of infection in the mortuary and post mortem room*, HMSO, London.

Health and Safety Executive (1995) *Categorisation of biological agents according to hazard and categories of containment*. Advisory Committee on Dangerous Pathogens, HMSO London.

HMSO (1995). Hospital laundry arrangements for used and infected linen, HSG(95)18, NHS Executive. HMSO, London.

Johnson, G. and Robinson, W. (1990) Human Immunodeficiency Virus (HIV–1) in vapours of surgical power instruments. *Journal of Medical Virology*, **33**, 47–56.

Kubler-Ross, E. (1982) *Living with Death and Dying*. Macmillan, London.

Newson, W., Rowlands, C., Matthews, J. and Elliot, C.J. (1983) Aerosols in the mortuary. *Journal of Clinical Pathology*, **36**, 127–32.

Philpott–Howard, J. and Casewell, M., (1994) *Hospital Infection Control Policies and Practical Procedures*. WB Saunders Co. Ltd, London.

Shanson, D.C. (Co-ordinator of Working Party) (1992) Risks to surgeons and patients from HIV and Hepatitis; guidelines on precautions and management of exposure to blood and body fluids. Joint Working Party of the Hospital Infection Society and the Surgical Infection Study Group. *British Medical Journal*, **305**, 1337–43.

Speck, P. (1992) Care after death. *Nursing Times*, **88**, (6).

Wright, J., Cousins, J. and Upward, J. (1988) *Matters of death and life – A study of bereavement support in NHS hospitals in England*. Project Paper, King's Fund Publishing Office, London.

Young, T. and Healing, T. (1995) Infection in the deceased; a survey of management. *CDR*, **5**, PHL, Review 5.

FURTHER READING

Caddow, P. (1989) *Applied Microbiology*. Scutari Press, London.

Department of Health (1991) *Decontamination of Equipment; Linen or other surfaces contaminated with Hepatitis B and or HIV*. Microbiology Advisory Committee, HMSO, London.

Green, J. (1991) *Death with dignity. Meeting the spiritual needs of patients in a multicultural society*. Nursing Times Book Service, Lincolnshire.

HMSO (1974) Health & Safety at Work Act, London.

Lowbury, E., Ayliffe, G.A.F., Geddes, A. and Williams, J. (1992) *Control of Infection in Hospital. A Practical Handbook*. Chapman & Hall, London.

Appendix A

LIST OF COMMUNICABLE DISEASES AND ISOLATION PRECAUTIONS

*Diseases marked * must be notified to the proper officer, usually the local CCDC by telephone*

Disease	Infective material	Isolation precautions	Duration of infectivity
AIDS	Blood and body fluids	Follow UICP	Indefinitely
Amoebiasis (N)	Faeces	Care with stool. No isolation required	Until stool negative on microscopy
Anthrax (N) (pulmonary)	Respiratory tract secretions	Strict isolation	Duration of illness
Anthrax (cutaneous)	Exudate from lesion	Standard isolation	Culture negative
Brucellosis	None	None	None
Campylobacter (R)	Faeces	Standard isolation	Duration of diarrhoea
Candidiasis	None	None	None
Chickenpox*	Respiratory secretions and skin lesions	Do not have contact unless history of chickenpox. Single room with door closed	At least 1 week from start of eruption. Wait until all lesions crusted
Chlamydia trachomatis eye genital	Discharges of exudate	None	Duration of illness
Chlamydia pneumonia	Respiratory secretions	Standard and mask	Duration of illness

Disease	Infective material	Isolation precautions	Duration of infectivity
Chlamydia psittaci (Psittacosis)	Respiratory secretions	None	Duration of illness. Very occasionally transmissible human to human if paroxysmal coughing
Cholera (N)	Faeces	Standard	Duration of diarrhoea
Clostridium difficile/Pseudo-membranous colitis/antibiotic associated colitis	Faeces	Standard	Duration of diarrhoea
Common cold	Oral secretions	No isolation	Duration of illness
Cryptosporidium (R)	Faeces	Standard	Duration of diarrhoea
Diarrhoea (unknown origin - presumed infective)	Faeces	Standard	Duration of diarrhoea
Diphtheria (N) (pharyngeal)	Nasal and/or oral secretions	Strict	Until nose and throat cultures negative
Diphtheria (N) (cutaneous)	Lesion Secretions	Standard	Duration of lesions
Dysentery (N)			*See*: food poisoning and specific causative organisms
Ebola virus (N)			*See*: viral haemorrhagic fever
Eczema vaccinatum vaccinia	Fluid from lesions	Strict	Until all crusts separated

Disease	Infective material	Isolation precautions	Duration of infectivity
Encephalitis viral (N)	Nasal and throat secretions	Standard	First few days of illness
Food poisoning causative agent often not known – treat as *Salmonella*	Faeces	Standard	Duration of diarrhoea (and/or vomiting)
Campylobacter (N)			
Staph. aureus (N)		None	
B. cereus (N)		None	
C. perfringens (N)		None	
C. botulinum (N)	Saliva, urine	None	
Gas gangrene *Clostridium perfringens*	Lesion secretions	None	
Giardiasis	Faeces	Standard	Duration of diarrhoea
Gonorrhoea and ophthalmia neonatorum (N)	Discharge	Standard – only required for infants	Until 24 hours of antibiotic treatment
Helminths		None	
Hepatitis A (N)	Faeces	Standard	In first seven days of illness
Hepatitis E	Faeces	Standard	
Hepatitis (?cause)	Faeces	Standard	Until disease identified
Hepatitis B (N)	Blood and body fluids	UICP	No isolation required if patients are not bleeding and are not likely to bleed
Hepatitis C (N)	Blood and body fluids	UICP	No isolation required if patients are not bleeding and are not likely to bleed

Disease	Infective material	Isolation precautions	Duration of infectivity
Herpes simplex (severe)	Lesion secretions	Standard	Until lesions have dried and crusted
Herpes zoster (shingles)*	Lesion secretions	As for chickenpox	Until lesions have crusted
HIV (AIDS)	Blood and body fluids	See AIDS	Indefinitely
Impetigo	Skin lesions	Standard	Duration of illness
Influenza	Oral secretions	Standard	Duration of illness
Lassa fever (N)		*See*: viral haemorrhagic fever	
Legionnaires' disease (R)	None		
Leprosy (N) smear positive	Lesions and nasal secretions	Standard	Duration of initial stay in hospital
Leprosy (N) Smear negative		None	
Leptospirosis (N)	Blood and urine	Urine precautions only	Until completion of treatment
Lice (head/body)	Hair/clothing	Standard	Until 24 hours after treatment
Malaria (N)		None	
Marburg (N)		*See*: viral haemorrhagic fever	
Measles (R)	Respiratory secretions/ droplets	Standard (to protect patient)	Five days after onset of rash
Meningitis bacterial (N) meningococcal	Oral secretions	Standard	Until 48 hours after antibiotic treatment.

Disease	Infective material	Isolation precautions	Duration of infectivity
			Eradication requires course of rifampicin (or ciprofloxacin) at the end of a suppressive course
Meningitis bacterial (N) Other bacterial	Oral secretions	Standard	Until 24 hours after antibiotic treatment
Meningitis viral (N)	Oral secretions faeces	Standard	Duration of illness
Mumps (N)		Standard	Duration of illness
Polio (N)		Standard	Duration of illness
Multi-resistant bacteria	Source, *e.g.* sputum, urine, stool, lesions	Standard	Seek advice from ICP
MRSA (methicillin resistant *Staphylococcus aureus*)	Lesions, skin, nose *etc.*	Standard	Seek advice from ICP
Mumps (N)	*Oral secretions urine	Standard	Until nine days after onset of parotid swelling
Ophthalmia neonatorum	Discharge	Standard	For first 24 hours of antibiotic treatment
Parvovirus B19			Not infectious once rash develops. Immuno-compromised patients may secrete virus for weeks/months

Disease	Infective material	Isolation precautions	Duration of infectivity
Pertussis (N) whooping cough	Oral secretions	Standard	Until seven days after start of treatment
Plague (N)		Strict	
Pneumococci	Respiratory secretions	None: standard if organism is resistant to penicillin	Nosocomial infection rare but has been recorded
Pneumocystis		None	
Poliomyelitis (N)	Faeces	Standard	Until 7 days after onset
Pseudomem-branous colitis		See: *Clostridium difficile*	
Psittacosis		See: *Chlamydia psittaci*	
Q Fever	Possible respiratory secretions	None	Low risk person to person spread. Only possibility pneumonia
Rabies (N)	Saliva	Seek immediate advice from CCDC/GP	Throughout clinical disease
Rashes	Possibly saliva or oral secretions or lesion fluids	Standard	Until diagnosis confirmed then adjust appropriately
Respiratory syncytial virus	Oral and respiratory secretions	Standard	Duration of illness (longer in immuno-compromised patients)
Ringworm, *Tinea pedis, Corporis, capitis*	Hair, skin, clothing	None	Duration of lesions
Rotavirus	Faeces	Standard	Duration of illness

Disease	Infective material	Isolation precautions	Duration of infectivity
Rubella (N) congenital	Urine and oral secretions	Standard. **N.B.** Staff must all be vaccinated and immunity proven prior to caring for children	Duration of hospital stay, for 1st year of life if hospitalised
Rubella, acquired (N)	Oral secretions	Standard	Until five days after onset of rash
Salmonella		See: food poisoning	
Scabies	Skin	Standard	For 24 hours after start of treatment
Shigella (N)	Faeces	Standard	Duration of illness
Staphylococcal infection (excluding MRSA)	Lesions	None unless shedding large amount of skin scales	
Streptococci			
Groups A, C and G pharyngitis,	Oral secretions	Standard	Until 48 hours after start of
scarlet fever (N) Puerperal fever Burns/wounds Cellulitis	Skin lesions	Standard	effective antibiotic therapy
Syphilis	Lesions	Standard	Until 24 hours after start of treatment
Tetanus (N)		None	
Toxoplasmosis		None	
Trichomoniasis	Vaginal discharge	None	
Tuberculosis (N) Pulmonary smear positive (open) Other cases	Sputum Ensure sputum negative	Standard/masks if necessary	Two weeks after start of effective treatment

Disease	Infective material	Isolation precautions	Duration of infectivity
Typhoid and Paratyphoid (N)	Faeces/urine	Standard	Duration of illness: three negative stools required for food handlers
Typhus	Skin lesions	Standard	Until de-lousing complete
Whooping Cough (N)		*See*: Pertussis	
Worms/ helminths	Usually faeces	None	
Viral Diarrhoea norwalk, calici, winter vomiting disease, small round structured virus	Faeces/vomit	Standard	Duration of diarrhoea, environmental contamination is very important in spread of disease
Viral haemorrhagic fever (N)	Blood and body secretions	Strict	Discuss with Infection Control Practitioner
Yellow Fever (N)		Standard	
Zoster		*See*: chickenpox shingles	

(N) Notifiable disease, if suspected report immediately to CCDC
(R) Reportable to CCDC
* Staff unable to give a definite history of having had relevant disease must not look after patient
** Should not be in ward with other immunocompromised patients

Appendix B

USEFUL ADDRESSES

Association for Practitioners in Infection Control and Epidemiology Inc. (APIC)
1016 16th Street NW
Sixth floor
Washington DC
20036 USA

001 202 296 2742

Association of Anaesthetists
9, Bedford Square
London
WC1B 3RA

0171 631 1650

Association of Medical Microbiologists
Secretary: Dr Peter Wilkinson
Public Health Laboratory
University Hospital
Queen's Medical Centre
Nottingham
NG7 2UH

01602 709161

BAPS
DSS Distribution Centre
Heywood Stores
Manchester Road
Heywood
Lancashire
OL10 2PZ

British Dental Association
64, Wimpole Street
London
W1M 8AL

0171 935 0875

Central Public Health Laboratory Service
61, Colindale Avenue
London
NW9 5HT

0181 200 4400

Department of Health
Richmond House
79, Whitehall
London
SW1A 2NS

0171 210 4850

Health & Safety Executive
Information Centre
Broad Lane
Sheffield
S3 7HQ

0114 289 2333

Infection Control Nurses Association
Honorary Secretary
Miss Gwen Davis
Dept. of Bacteriology
John Radcliffe Hospital
Headington
Oxford
OX3 9DU

Institute of Environmental Health Officers
Chadwick Court
15, Hatfields
London
SE1 8DJ

0171 928 6006

King's Fund Centre
126, Albert Street
London
NW1 7NF

0171 267 6111

Medical Devices Directorate
14, Russell Square
London
WC1B 5EP

Adverse Incident Reporting:
Helpline: 0171 972 8100/1/2
Hotline: 0171 972 8080

Public Health Medicine Environmental Group
Secretary Dr R. Buttery
Public Health Medicine
Cambridge Health Authority
Ferndale Offices
(366) Fulbourn Hospital
Fulbourn
Cambridge
CB1 5EF

01223 218843

Wound Care Society
PO Box 263
Northampton
NN3 4UJ

Appendix C

GLOSSARY AND ABBREVIATIONS

ACDP	Advisory Committee on Dangerous Pathogens
Acquired immunity	Immunity which develops as the result of a stimulus, e.g. an infection
Aerobe	An organism that grows in the presence of oxygen
AFB	Acid fast bacilli
Agar	A polysaccharide made from seaweed and used in bacteriological media
AHA	Area Health Authority
AIDS	Acquired immune deficiency syndrome
Algae	Photosynthetic organisms
Anaerobe	An organism that grows in the absence of oxygen
Antibiotic	A substance which is toxic to certain organisms
Antibody	A protein which appears in an animal after contact with an antigen
Antigen	A substance which an animal's body regards as foreign and produces antibodies against
APIC	Association for Professionals in Infection Control and Epidemiology
ATP	Adenosine triphosphate
Autoclave	A machine in which instruments etc. are exposed to steam under pressure
Bacillus	A rod shaped bacterium
Bacteraemia	Bacteria in the blood
Bacteria	Plural of bacterium
Bactericidal	Capable of killing bacteria
Bacteriostatic	Inhibit or slow growth of bacteria, but not kill
Bacterium	Any prokaryotic organism. They are single celled micro-organims that differ from all other organisms (the eukaryotes) in lacking a true nucleus and organelles
Barrier nursing	A form of isolation nursing
BSE	Bovine spongiform encephalitis
BSI	Body substance isolation

CAMO	Chief Administration Officer
CAPD	Continuous ambulatory peritoneal dialysis
Capsule	An enclosing structure
Carrier	An individual who persistently excretes a microbe or whose body is colonised with a microbe, but who does not exhibit signs of infection
Catheter	A tubular flexible instrument passed through body channels for withdrawal or introduction of fluids
CCDC	Consultant in communicable disease control
CDC	Center for disease control and prevention
CDCP	Centers for disease control and prevention
CDR	Communicable disease report
CDSC	Communicable disease surveillance centre
CECHC	Chief executive community health council
Chlamydia	A genus of bacteria comprising two species
Chloroplasts	The photosynthetic unit of a plant cell, containing all the chlorophyll
Chromosome	A structure in the nucleus (of animal cells) containing a linear thread of DNA which transmits genetic material
CICN	Community infection control nurse
CJD	Creutzfeld–Jakob disease
CMO	Chief medical officer
CNO	Chief nursing officer
Colonisation	A microbe which establishes itself in a particular environment without producing disease or symptoms
Commensal	An organism which lives in association with another without benefiting or harming it.
Communicable	A disease that can be transmitted from one person to another
Community acquired infection	An infection acquired while the person was in the community, not hospital
Contagious	As communicable
COSHH	Control of Substances Hazardous to Health Regulations
CPHL	Central Public Health Laboratory
CPHM	Consultant in public health medicine
Cross infection	Infection transmitted between patients infected with pathogenic micro-organims
CSSD	Central Sterile Supply Department
CSU	Catheter specimen of urine
Culture	The propagation of micro-organisms or of living cells in special media conducive to their growth
Cytoplasm	The protoplasm of a cell surrounding the nucleus

Decontamination	To remove a contaminating substance from an object or person
Deoxyribonucleic acid (DNA)	A nucleic acid of complex molecular structure occurring in cell nuclei as the basic structure of the genes
DHA	District Health Authority
DHSS	Department of Health and Social Services
DICC	District infection control committee
Disinfect	To destroy micro-organisms but not usually bacterial spores, reducing the number of micro-organims to a level which is not harmful to health
Disinfectant	An agent, usually a chemical, which destroys infection producing micro-organisms
Disinfection	The act of disinfecting
DM(DFM)	Dust-mist (Dust-fume mist)
DoE	Department of the Environment
DoH	Department of Health
EHO	Environmental Health Officer
EL	Executive letter
Electron	Negatively charged atomic particle, one of three types of particle that make up the atom
Electron microscope	A type of microscope (first developed in 1930s) giving high magnification and resolution by employing a beam of electrons instead of light
ELISA	Enzyme linked immunosorbent assay
Endemic	A disease or infection constantly present in the community
Endogenous	Growing or originating from within
Endoplasmic reticulum	A complicated membrane system extending throughout the cytoplasm of a eukaryotic cell
Endoscope	An instrument used for direct visual inspection of hollow organs of the body
Endotoxin	A heat stable toxin present in the intact bacterial cell but not in cell free filtrates or cultures of intact bacteria
Endotracheal tube	An airway catheter inserted into the trachea during endotracheal intubation
Entamoeba	A genus of parasitic amoebas in the intestines of invertebrates
Enteric	Pertaining to the small intestine
Enterobacter	A genus of bacteria
Enzyme	A protein that acts as a catalyst, increasing the rate at which a chemical reaction occurs
EPI	Extended programme on immunisation

Epidemic	The presence in a population of disease or infection in excess of that usually expected
Epidemiologist	An expert in epidemiology
Epidemiology	The study of the distribution of factors determining health and disease in human populations, and in the application of this study to the prevention and control of disease
Epidermis	The outermost and nonvascular layer of the skin
Epithelium	The cellular covering of internal and external surfaces of the body
Epstein–Barr virus	A herpes virus that is the aetiological agent of infectious mononucleosis
Erysipelas	A febrile disease characterised by inflammation and redness of the skin and subcutaneous tissues due to Group A haemolytic streptococci
Erythema	Redness of the skin caused by congestion of the capillaries in the lower layers of the skin
Erythrocyte	A red blood cell, or corpuscle
Escherichia	A genus of widely distributed Gram-negative bacteria
Eukaryotic cell	A cell with a true nucleus bounded by a nuclear membrane, and containing chromosomes which divide by mitosis
Exogenous	Originating outside or caused by factors outside the organism
Exotoxin	A potent toxin formed and excreted by the bacterial cell
Exposure	The condition of being subjected to something infectious
Fertilisation	Process by which the male's sperm unites with the female's ovum
FHSA	Family Health Service Authority
Fibreoptic (endoscope)	A flexible endoscope whose lumen is coated with fibreoptic glass or plastic fibres with special optical properties
Flagellate	Any micro-organism having flagells
Flagellum	A long, mobile, whip like appendage arising from a basal body at the surface of a cell, serving as a locomotor organelle
Flora (normal)	Bacteria usually residing on the body of man, without harming man
Fomites	Inanimate objects or materials on which disease producing agents may be conveyed
FPC	Family Practitioner Committee

Gene	One of the biological units of heredity, self-reproducing and located at a definite position on a particular chromosome
Generic	Non-proprietary; denoting a drug name not protected by a trademark
Genus	A taxonomic category (taxon) subordinate to a tribe (or subtribe) and superior to a species (or subgenus)
Giardia	A genus of flagellate protozoa parasitic in the intestines of man and animals, which may cause protracted diarrhoea
Gonococcus	An individual of the species *Neiserria gonorrhoeae*
GP	General practioner
Gram's stain	A staining procedure in which bacteria are stained with crystal violet, treated with strong iodine solution, decolourized with ethanol or ethanol–acetone, and counterstained with a contrasting dye; those retaining the stain are Gram-positive, those losing the stain but staining with the counterstain are Gram-negative
Gram-negative	*See Gram's stain*
Gram-positive	*See Gram's stain*
Guanine	A purine base, one of the fundamental components of nucleic acids (DNA and RNA)
Guinea worm	A nematode worm
HA	Health authority
HAI	Hospital acquired infection, an infection acquired during hospitalisation or as a result of hospital treatment
HAV	Hepatitis A virus
HBeAg	Hepatitis B e antigen
HBIG	Hepatitis B immune globulin
HBsAg	Hepatitis B surface antigen
HBV	Hepatitis B virus
HC	Health circular
HCV	Hepatitis C virus
HCW	Health care worker
HEPA	High efficiency particulate air
Hepatitis	Inflammation of the liver; there are many causes of hepatitis, many are viruses
HICC	Hospital infection control committee
HIV	Human immunodeficiency virus
HSAWA	Health and Safety at Work Act
HSDU	Hospital sterilisation and decontamination unit
HSE	Health and Safety Executive
HSG	Health service guidelines

HV	Health visitor
Hydrophobic	Repelling water, insoluble in water, not readily absorbing water
Hydrophylic	Having strongly polar groups which readily interact with water
ICC	Infection control committee
ICD	Infection control doctor
ICLN	Infection control link nurses
ICN	Infection control nurse
ICNA	Infection control nurses association
ICO	Infection control officers
ICP	Infection control practitioner
ICT	Infection control team
Immune	Being highly resistant to a disease due to the formation of humoral antibodies, the development of immunological competent cells, or both or as the result of another mechanism
Immunity	The condition of being immune, either through prior infection or immunisation
Immunisation	The process of rendering a subject immune, or of becoming immune
Immunoglobulin	A protein of animal origin with known antibody activity
Incidence	The number of new events/diseases which occur in a population in a given time period
Incubation (period)	The interval between the entrance of the pathogen and the development of symptoms. Will vary from pathogen to pathogen
Infection	Invasion and multiplication of micro-organisms in body tissues, particularly those causing local cellular injury due to competitive metabolism, toxins, intracellular replication or antigen-antibody response
Infectious	Caused by or capable of being communicated by infection
Inflammation	A localized protective response elicited by injury or destruction of tissues, characterised by swelling, heat, redness and pain which serves to destroy, dilute or wall off both the injurious agent and the injured tissue
Intracellular	Inside cells
Intravascular (device)	Catheter/cannula inserted into a vein or artery
Isolation precautions	Additional precautions to be taken with some patients/clients/residents
Klebsiella	A genus of Gram-negative bacteria

LA	Local authority
Lassa Fever	A viral haemorrhagic fever
Listeria	A genus of Gram-negative bacteria
Lysosomes	Minute membrane bound vacuoles occurring in many types of cells
MAFF	Ministry of Agriculture, Fisheries and Food
MDRTB	Multi-drug resistant tuberculosis
Meiosis	The process of cell division by which reproductive cells, gametes, are formed
Meningitis	Inflammation of the meninges, two common causes: bacterial and viral
Metabolism	The sum of the physical and chemical processes by which a living organised substance is built up and maintained.
Microorganism	A microscopic organism
MIC	Minimum inhibitory concentration
Mitochondria	Small, spherical to rod shaped membrane bounded cytoplasmic organelles which are the principle site of the ATP synthesis
Mitosis	The ordinary process of cell division, which results in the formation of two identical daughter cells
MMWR	Morbidity and Mortality Weekly Report
MOH	Medical officer of health
MRSA	Methicillin resistant *Staphylococcus aureus*
Mycobacterium	A genus of gram-positive bacteria characterised by acid fast staining
Mycology	The study of fungi and fungus
Mycoplasma	A genus of highly pleomorphic Gram-negative aerobic bacteria
Mycosis	Any disease caused by fungi
MOCG	Major outbreak control group
MOEH	Medical Officer of Environmental Health
MSU	Midstream specimen of urine
NHS	National Health Service
NHSE	National Health Service Executive
NHSME	National Health Service Management Executive
Nosocomial	Hospital acquired (infection)
Nucleolus	A rounded refractile body in the nucleus of most cells
Nucleus	In a cell, a spheroid body containing the chromosomes and one or more nucleoli
Obligate	An organism which can only survive in one type of environment, or assumes only one particular role
OCG	Outbreak control group

ONS	Office of National Statistics, formerly OPCS
Opportunistic	A micro-organism which does not normally cause disease but becomes pathogenic under certain circumstances
Organelle	A specialised structure of a cell such as a mitochondrion, Golgi apparatus
OSHA	Occupational Safety and Health Administration
Outbreak	An incident in which two or more people have the same disease, similar symptoms or excrete the same patho-gens, and in which there is a time/place/person association. Also a situation where the observed number of cases unaccountably exceeds the expected number
Pandemic	A widespread epidemic disease, over a wide area worldwide
Parasite	A plant or animal which lives upon or within another living organism, at whose expense it gains some advantage
Passive immunity	Immunity conferred on the host by antibodies made in another host
Pathogen	Any disease producing agent or micro-organism
Pathogenesis	The processes involved in the development of disease
Pathogenicity	The quality of producing or the ability to produce pathological changes or disease
PCP	*Pneumocystis carinii* pneumonia
Penicillin	Any of a large group of natural or semi-synthetic antibacterial antibiotics derived directly or indirectly from strains of fungi of the genus *Penicillum*
Peptide	Any of a class of compounds of low molecular weight which yield two or more amino acids on hydrolysis
pH	The means by which a solution is measured to be either acidic or alkaline (0–14), a low pH is acidic, a high pH alkaline
Phage (typing)	Characterisation of bacteria. Parasitic viruses attach to some bacteria and are used to subdivide strains with a particular serotype
Phagocyte	Any cell that ingests micro-organisms or other cells and foreign particles
Phagocytosis	The engulfing of micro-organisms or other cells and foreign bodies by phagocytes
PHLS	Public Health Laboratory Service
PHMEG	Public Health Medicine Environmental Group
Phospholipid	Any lipid that contains phosphorus

Photosynthesis	A chemical combination caused by the action of light, specifically the formation of carbohydrates from carbon dioxide and water in the chlorophyll tissue of plants under the influence of light
Plasma	The fluid portion of blood
Plasmid	Any extrachromosomal self-replicating genetic element of a cell
Plasmodium	A genus of sporozoa parasitic in the red blood cells of man, the malarial parasite
Pneumococcus	An individual of the species *Streptococcus pneumoniae*, the commonest cause of lobar pneumonia
Prevalence	The total number of cases of a specific disease in existence in a given population at a certain time
Prokaryotic cell	A unicellular organism lacking a true nucleus and nuclear membrane, having genetic material composed of a single loop of naked double stranded DNA
Prophylaxis	Preventative treatment
Protective isolation	A type of isolation designed to protect the immuno-compromised patient from infections from other patients and HCWs
Protozoa	Unicelluar eukaryotic organisms, mostly free living
PHLS	Public Health Laboratory Service
Puerperal fever	An infectious disease of childbirth
Purulence	The formation or presence of pus
Pus	A protein rich liquid inflammation product
RAWP	Resource Allocation Working Party
Replication	Viral multiplication
Reproduction	The process by which a living entity or organism produces a new individual of the same kind
RHA	Regional Health Authority
Ribonucleic acid (RNA)	A nucleic acid present in all living cells which controls cellular protein synthesis and replaces DNA as a carrier of genetic codes in some viruses
Ribosome	Any of the intracellular ribonucleoprotein particles concerned with protein synthesis
Rickettsia	A genus of small rod shaped to round micro-organisms found in the cytoplasm of tissue cells of lice, fleas, ticks and mites, and passed to man by their bites
RIDDOR	Reporting of Injuries, Diseases and Dangerous Occurrences Regulations
Saprophyte	An organism such as a bacterium living on dead or decaying organic matter
Serology	The study of antigen–antibody reactions *in vitro*

Serotype	The type of a microorganism determined by its constituent antigens, or a taxonomic subdivision
Species	A taxonomic category subordinate to a genus, and superior to a subspecies
Spore	An oval body formed within bacteria which is regarded as a resting stage during the life cycle of the cell; it is characterized by its resistance to environmental changes
Sterilisation	The process of destroying or removing all living microorganisms
Surveillance	Observation of the occurrence of disease in a population, with analysis and dissemination of the results
TB	Tuberculosis
T Cell	One of the two main cell types of the immune system responsible for cell-mediated immunity
Toxin	Any poisonous substance produced by a living organism
Toxoid	A toxin treated by heat or chemical agent to destroy its deleterious properties without destroying its ability to combine with or stimulate the formation of antitoxin
UICP	Universal infection control precautions
Unicellular	Made up of one single cell, as bacteria
UTI	Urinary tract infection
Vaccination	The introduction of vaccine into the body to produce immunity to a specific disease
Vaccine	A suspension of attenuated or killed micro-organisms (viruses, bacteria or rickettsiae) administered for the prevention, amelioration, or treatment of infectious disease
VRE	Vancomycin resistant enterococci
VHF	Viral haemorrhagic fever
Virulence	The degree of pathogenicity of a micro-organism as indicated by case fatality rates and/or its ability to invade the tissues of the host
Virus	Any member of a unique class of infectious agents
WDA	Waste Disposal Authority
WHO	World Health Organisation
WRA	Waste regulation authority
Yeast	A general term including unicellular nucleated, usually rounded fungi

Index

Page numbers printed in **bold** type refer to figures; those in *italic* to tables. Individual items in the glossary (pages 214–23) are not indexed.

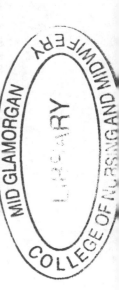